Comfort
at Your
Computer

Comfort
at Your
Computer

**Body
Awareness
Training
for
Pain-Free
Computer Use**

Paul Linden, Ph.D.

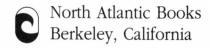
North Atlantic Books
Berkeley, California

Published by

North Atlantic Books

P.O. Box 12327

Berkeley, California 94712

Cover and book design by Nancy Koerner

Printed in the United States of America

Comfort at Your Computer was originally published by Prentice Hall, Inc. under the title *Compute in Comfort: Body Awareness Training: A Day-to-Day Guide to Pain-Free Computing.*

Comfort at Your Computer is sponsored by the Society for the Study of Native Arts and Sciences, a nonprofit educational corporation whose goals are to develop an educational and crosscultural perspective linking various scientific, social, and artistic fields; to nurture a holistic view of arts, sciences, humanities, and healing; and to publish and distribute literature on the relationship of mind, body, and nature.

Library of Congress Cataloging-in-Publication Data

Linden, Paul.

      Comfort at your computer : body awareness training for pain-free
computer use : a practical guide / Paul Linden.

        p.   cm.

     ISBN 1-55643-322-0 (alk. paper)

     1. Overuse injuries--Prevention. 2. Computers--Health aspects.

  I. Title.

RC965.V53L558 1999

613.6'2--ds21   99-16526

                                   CIP

1 2 3 4 5 6 7 8 9 / 05 04 03 02 01 00

DEDICATION

Now I know why authors in their dedications always thank their families for putting up with them while they wrote their books. It's because for a whole year they were obsessed with their books, spending all day and all night at their computers, and never washing the dishes. So, thank you Peggy and Joshua for being my family and for putting up with me while I wrote my book.

TABLE OF CONTENTS

PART I—YOUR BODY

1—THE COMPUTER PROBLEM **3**
>   *Body Awareness:*
>   *A New Way of Approaching the Problem*
>   *How to use the book*
>   *Scope of the book*

2—BODY AWARENESS IS THE KEY **13**
>   *Body Awareness*
>   *Holism*

3—WHAT IS COMPUTER STRESS? **25**
>   *What is stress?*
>   *General effects of computer stress*
>   *Identifying stress*
>   *Musculoskeletal aspects of stress*
>   *Causes of stress in computer work*

4—SOFTENING YOUR BREATHING AND VOICE **51**

5—BALANCING YOUR PELVIS AND
SPINAL COLUMN **71**

6—GETTING TO THE HEART OF IT **87**

7—GAINING EASE IN YOUR HANDS,
ARMS AND SHOULDERS **93**

8—IMPROVING USE OF YOUR LEGS **109**

9—RELAXING AND BALANCING YOUR
HEAD AND NECK **129**

10—USING YOUR EYES COMFORTABLY **137**

11—WHAT GOOD SITING POSTURE IS AND IS NOT **153**

12—FIVE-SECOND MOVEMENT BREAKS
   DURING WORK **165**

13—TWENTY-MINUTE MOVEMENT SESSIONS
   FOR HOME **181**

14—THREE-MINUTE MOVEMENT BREAKS
   FOR THE OFFICE **199**

PART II—YOUR WORK ENVIRONMENT

15—MAKING YOUR DESKTOP WORKSTATION

   COMFORTABLE **209**
   General points
   Chair
   Desk
   Input devices
   Monitor
   Paper documents

16—USING LAPTOPS **255**
   Using your laptop
   On an airplane
   Laptops with trackballs
   Carrying your laptop

17—STANDING WORKSTATION **281**

18—CHANGING THE WORK ENVIRONMENT **291**

19—THE BEGINNING **297**

APPENDIX A—
   WORKSHOPS AND CONSULTATIONS **301**

APPENDIX B—
   QUESTIONS AND COMMENTS **303**

APPENDIX C—
   BIOGRAPHY **305**

INDEX **307**

ACKNOWLEGDMENTS

I owe Dawn Costick special thanks for her imagination and skill in doing the photography. She is a massage therapist as well as a photographer, and her ability to see the body in both ways was invaluable in organizing the visual presentation of the book and shooting the photographs.

Tom Simpson contributed a lot to the book. He coaxed me into getting my first computer, way back when, and he generously took time to serve as a model for the photographs—in which he demonstrated with great clarity body intelligence in movement.

Raphael Rosado took my jokes and turned them into cartoons that are each worth more than a thousand words.

Nancy Sally prepared the anatomical drawings, and Gail Griffith served as a model in the photographs.

Barbara Braham, an author and public speaker, gave me valuable advice on the book and listened to my ongoing reports on how far the writing had come.

Marilyn Huheey was kind enough to review the chapters on head and eyes. Barbara Fredin, Jean Pierre Dujardin, Russell Hall, and David Berger all read the manuscript and offered detailed critiques that were immensely helpful.

Aikido gave me my appreciation of the body in movement. I am grateful for the existence of Aikido, and I am grateful to all my practice partners down through the years and to all the instructors who have helped me progress in the art, especially Robert Nadeau and Yoshimitsu Yamada.

I owe all my students through the years a debt of gratitude. I learned by teaching them.

I appreciate the help that Keri Walker at Apple Computer and Aida Adams at Communication Intelligence Corporation each extended in arranging for me to try out pieces of equipment.

Special thanks are due to the people at Feldenkrais Resources, who thought this book should stay available and who brought it to the attention of North Atlantic Books. And special thanks are due to Richard Grossinger at North Atlantic who found the book worth republishing.

COMFORT
AT YOUR COMPUTER LITE

Comfort at Your Computer covers a lot of material. For those of you who are in a hurry, or for those of you who wish to conduct a brief, basic computer safety course at your workplace or school, this is a listing of the key sections of the book to read and practice for comfortable, safe use of a desktop computer. (For information about laptops and standing workstations, you could add material from the chapters on those topics.)

Reading these few sections about the basics of appropriate computer use will do a lot to help you start getting more comfortable at your computer right away. However, much of the usefulness of *Comfort at Your Computer* lies in the richness of detail provided in the rest of the book. For information on how to solve specific problems, consult the appropriate sections in the book. For a more complete understanding of how to work safely at your computer, when you have time work through the rest of the material in the book.

YOUR BODY

Body Awareness, pages 3–11
Body Awareness Experiments, pages 13–21
Stress, pages 25–28, 32–35
Breathing and Voice, pages 51–53, 58, 61–69
Pelvic Balance, pages 76–79
Towel Sitting, pages 82–83
Chest, pages 87–88
Hands and Arms, pages 99–101
Head and Eyes, pages 132–133, 140
Movement Breaks, pages 165–179

YOUR WORKSTATION

Chair, pages 213–221

Desk, pages 221–225

Keyboard, pages 225–226

Mouse, pages 231–232

Monitor, pages 243–247

PART I

YOUR BODY

THE COMPUTER PROBLEM

Spending long hours at a computer keyboard can hurt. Many people experience pain in their eyes, neck, arms, hands, back or legs. Many people experience stress and anxiety. At best, this reduces concentration and productivity. At worst, it leads to serious physical damage.

People use computers in many different situations. Some people use the computer for entertainment and others use computers for work. There are individuals who use computers at home. There are individuals who work alone or in small offices. There are people who work in schools, universities or large companies. And of course children and students use computers both at home and at school. Everyone who uses computers should pay attention to issues of work comfort and safety, and parents and teachers should make sure that the young people in their care do not develop computer-related injuries.

Computer stress and repetitive motion injuries lead to a tremendous loss of productivity and a great deal of money being spent on medical treatment and litigation. People with serious computer-related injuries may have to stop using computers altogether. Students may find it very hard to do school work, and people in the workforce may find themselves unemployed and unemployable.

But life with a computer doesn't have to hurt. It really can be surprisingly quick and easy to learn how to achieve a safe and comfortable way of working at your computer. *Comfort at Your Computer* will show you how to:
- work at your computer in a mentally and physically alert, relaxed and strain-free manner
- set up your computer workstation so that it enhances your comfort and productivity
- organize a computer-safety program at your school or workplace.

3

By gaining a greater understanding of the human body and the computer workstation, you will be able to:
• avoid computer stress and injuries
• choose proper workstation equipment
• save money on equipment
• reduce medical bills and lost work time
• increase job satisfaction and productivity.

Comfort at Your Computer will help you find simple, low-cost solutions that are easy to put into practice and take very little time.

The book presents the material in a personal, experiential format. Even if your main objective is to set up a computer safety program for your school or workplace, going through the body awareness exercises yourself will be the best way to understand the material and learn to teach it to others.

The best time to deal with computer stress and injuries is before they happen. Learning about relaxation, postural balance, and proper workstation setup will help you prevent computer-related problems. But if you are already experiencing problems, the same techniques for relieving computer stress will be helpful (along with proper medical treatment) in your recovery and in preventing future problems.

BODY AWARENESS:
A NEW WAY OF THINKING ABOUT THE PROBLEM

Computer-related injuries result from long hours of holding awkward, strained positions and from the repetitive movements of pounding keys. Before the advent of computers, office workers did not sit for hours in one fixed posture repeating the same few movements over and over again. Even using a typewriter, which is similar to using a computer, involved many different movements. Inserting paper, erasing mistakes, filing paper copies and so on forced typists to vary their movements. Computer users can sit for hours doing nothing but punching keys and staring at a screen.

Working at a computer for long hours is an intense and strenuous athletic event. Every athletic activity requires proper physical form and good equipment. If, for example, you jog with bad form and poor shoes, you weaken your performance and increase your risks of injury. Neither good form nor good equipment by itself is enough. In the same way, using a computer demands effective movement technique and good equipment.

Using effective movement technique means knowing what movements are required for the safest, most effective performance of the specific sport or task you are undertaking. *Effective movement technique starts with knowing your body.*

You have to know how to use your pelvis, legs and spinal column for sitting; your arms for typing; your head and eyes for looking at paper copy and the monitor; and your voice for dictation software. If you use a computer or video display terminal while standing up, you also need an awareness of the body mechanics of proper standing.

Proper equipment selection and workstation setup also start with knowing your body. Your furniture and workstation should support your body in your unique individual position of comfort. Your equipment must be able to adapt to your needs rather than forcing you to adapt to it. To pick out office furniture that fulfills your body's needs, you must know what your specific needs are.

Recommendations for safe computer-use are often given in terms of statistics about average body dimensions and general furniture requirements. However, you can't depend on statistics to tell you what your needs are. You can't depend on rules about what ought to be comfortable for the average person. You have to know what your own body actually needs for comfort. Once you can *feel*, in your own body and for yourself, when furniture actually does meet your needs, you will be able to judge when a piece of furniture is right for you.

Good equipment by itself is not enough. A bad chair will make good, comfortable sitting posture difficult if not impossible. But even a good chair won't help much if you are abusing your body through muscular tension and awkward posture. Sitting right on the wrong chair won't work, and sitting wrong on the right chair won't make you comfortable either. *Effective movement technique and proper equipment are both necessary in order to use a computer in comfort.*

In this book, I will concentrate on helping you learn how to think and feel for yourself. You will learn how to feel what will keep you safe and comfortable as you work at your computer. Once you can *feel* your body clearly, you won't sit and work in awkward, dangerous postures and you won't keep using uncomfortable and dangerous furniture. You will notice when something is hurtful to your body, and you will do something about it right away.

Most people have never thought about the need for body awareness training. Many people feel that if they can walk and talk and do all their other daily activities, they must already be aware of their bodies and know how to use them well.

Nothing could be farther from the truth. Many people can cope with ordinary, non-demanding activities, but hurt themselves as soon as they do something complicated or strenuous. Even small imbalances that would seem utterly harmless can, in the long run, add up to significant strain. Since working at a computer is both complex and strenuous, you need especially good body awareness and movement. If you don't use your body well, you will hurt yourself.

Computer stress can be prevented, and body awareness is the key.

HOW TO USE THIS BOOK

Comfort at Your Computer is organized very simply:

Part I: Your Body

Chapters 1–2: Introduction to the book; the nature of computer stress and its effects.

Chapters 3–11: A tour of your body, part by part, to help you experience and understand what comfort really is.

Chapters 12–14: Different movement and relaxation breaks.

Part II: Your Work

Chapters 15–17: How to set up your workstation and work environment for greatest comfort and safety.

Chapters 18–19: Changing the work environment; some final thoughts.

Much of *Comfort at Your Computer* will consist of body and movement awareness experiments and exercises. (Yes, I know. The word "exercises" and the idea of doing anything with the body remind many people of how much they hated gym class. Don't worry. These body awareness exercises will be totally different. They will be simple, easy and interesting. And no one will make fun of you for not knowing something. You can enjoy the movement experiments and be proud of yourself for wanting to learn.)

Most of the exercises you will do only once. They are *experiments* designed to increase your awareness of your body and your computer. Once you have done one of them, you will have felt and noticed something new that will be part of your awareness anytime you use your computer. Some of the exercises will be labeled as *practices* rather than experiments. In addition to being ways of learning new information, they are specific exercises that you can continue to practice on a long-term basis.

Most of the exercises will take very little time to do. Four or five minutes will be enough for each one, with only a few exceptions. Just by spending a few minutes at a time paying attention to your movements, you will be able to make startling changes in your comfort level.

It may be stating the obvious, but you will derive the greatest benefit from *doing* the exercises rather than just reading through them. Reading them will convey information, but doing them will develop *skill*. Gaining new information about how to sit and how to set up your workstation will certainly be helpful, but it is through developing practical skills in using your body properly that you will truly be able to use computers in comfort.

Every person is unique. People have different learning styles and different needs for information, explanations and practice. Some people will want to get right to the body awareness exercises, and others will want a clear intellectual introduction before they start. By the same token, readers using computers in a corporate environment will have different issues and needs than readers using computers at home. However, a book is a one-size-fits-all endeavor. Therefore, I have tried to balance different ways of presenting the material. But if some sections of *Comfort at Your Computer* don't really speak to you, just remember they probably speak to someone else, and keep reading.

You can go through the exercises in Part I at whatever pace works best for you. You could do a chapter each day. Or you might want to go more slowly, doing just one or two exercises a day. This would allow you to do all the exercises with minimal interruption of your work schedule. As long as spreading out the exercises does not destroy their coherence for you, a slower pace is fine. Since each chapter builds on the chapters before, you will find it most helpful to do the chapters in the order they are presented.

Why have I separated the tour of the body from the consideration of workstation set up? It might seem that consideration of the monitor, for example, should be in the section on eye use. The reason that I have organized the book this way is that a more holistic way of thinking is necessary for learning to work in comfort. It is true that you look at your monitor with your eyes. However, the way you use your eyes is related to how you position your head, which is dependent on, and also affects, how you organize your back, which in turn depends on and affects how you position your pelvis, which is strongly affected by how you use your legs. In other words, everything in the body forms an interlocking interconnected system.

When you examine any one element of your workstation, you have to consider every element of your body. In this book, first you will learn about your body, and then you will put that knowledge to use in organizing your workstation.

Please resist the temptation to jump right to the material on how to organize your workstation or to the sections on movement breaks that can be done while at the computer. Those sections of the book depend on the understanding and skill you will gain by doing and feeling the exercises in the initial chapters on body awareness.

You might enjoy doing these exercises in a small group, perhaps with people taking turns reading the instructions for the exercises and acting as leaders. It could be more fun doing the exercises with others, and it might provide better structure and motivation.

The most realistic practice of the material in this book will lie in putting the body awareness skills to work in your actual daily activities. However, don't get fanatical about maintaining "perfect posture." Learning to work comfortably at a computer may require a lot of changes in your style of body use. It will take a little time for those changes to become normal parts of your movement. And until they become so normal that they don't take any conscious attention to maintain, you will find yourself slipping into and out of new, more comfortable ways of working. Make sure not to tense yourself to hold onto your new, more relaxed sitting posture.

Getting compulsive about perfection will itself be stressful and will undermine your learning and progress. The best way to cultivate a new way of using your body will be to focus conscious attention on the new process for just a while and then let go of it. Later on, after you've let your "awareness batteries" recharge, you can go back to focusing on the new body pattern. This is important: you will fatigue yourself if you try to maintain continuous, permanent conscious attention to new physical processes. It will be so fatiguing that you will give up. Remember to pace yourself. Do a little every day, and as your awareness gets stronger, you will be able to do more and more.

Give yourself the gift of approaching your awareness training in a relaxed way. After all, it wouldn't make much sense to get all uptight about relaxation exercises, would it?

Give yourself the gift of patience and continuing curiosity. Discovering how to work in comfort is an ongoing *process* of learning. Finding comfort is not a once-and-for-all thing. As you begin to work with the exercises in this book, you will make changes right away that will vastly improve your comfort as you work at your computer. But as you continue to pay attention to noticing and feeling your body as you work, you will learn more. Your awareness of comfort and body use will change over time, and you will wish to change and improve what had already been a change for the better.

Even after you have worked your way through all the exercises in the book and put it away, it will be useful to open up the book once in a while and go through the exercises. That will help you refresh your memory of them and make sure you are still using them in your everyday work.

As you read more widely about the topics of body use and workstation design, you will find people advocating many different things. My advice is to adopt an experimental attitude, and my effort in this book is to give you enough information to enable you to make informed decisions. Try things out and decide for yourself what works for you. Adapt material to your own unique needs. Focus on what works for you and leave the rest.

SCOPE OF THE BOOK

There is much that is important in maintaining comfort at the computer and overall health that is outside the scope of this book. Consider examining other areas of health and wellness. Physical exercise is important. Sitting and typing for long periods is a very strenuous activity, and if you are in good physical shape, your muscles will have the strength and endurance to enable you to work comfortably at your computer. You also have to be well-rested to work effectively. If you are not rested, you won't have the energy to sit up properly or to focus mentally, so good sleep and recreation habits are important. Other areas of wellness such as not smoking, avoiding drug and alcohol use, eating healthfully, maintaining satisfying interpersonal relationships, and attending to the spiritual elements of human life are important as well. All these areas of awareness are part of overall health and work effectiveness, but this book focuses specifically on relaxation, physical flexibility, efficiency of posture, and workstation setup.

Comfort at Your Computer focuses primarily on the immediate workstation—the chair, the desk, and the computer—rather than the overall office environment. There is much information available about lighting, air quality, noise levels, office and building design, computer interface design, and so on. Those topics are certainly very relevant to the subject of computer stress, and some information will be included in this book, but a full treatment of them is outside its scope.

Comfort at Your Computer focuses on how to resolve problems of computer strain through more intelligent use of your body and more appropriate workstation setup. The book will concentrate on how to use common hardware rather than recommending solutions that depend on getting new or unusual keyboards or other esoteric hardware. Unusual equipment might be valuable, but there are two reasons for focusing on body awareness solutions. First and most important, equipment comes and goes, but the human body and the underlying principles of effective human movement stay the same. I don't know what currently available equipment will disappear or what kind of new equipment will be released after this book is published, but by focusing on how to feel what makes equipment good or bad, *Comfort at Your Computer* will give you a basis for judging the worth of anything you run across.

Another reason to focus on body awareness solutions is that getting new equipment can be expensive. Very often, finding more intelligent ways to use your body will reduce or eliminate computer stress without the need for spending money on new equipment. In only a few instances will this book mention specific kinds of hardware.

This book is not meant to take the place of proper medical diagnosis and treatment for those people with computer-related injuries or medical problems—though learning how to use your body in a safe and strain-free manner is a crucial and often neglected complement to medical treatment. If you are experiencing pain, numbness, or other physical difficulties from using your computer, it is very important to get appropriate medical treatment and not let the problem get worse. It would be most helpful to work with a physician who is knowledgeable about computer use, as well as body mechanics and movement, or who could refer you to an occupational or physical therapist with such knowledge.

This book focuses on what the average person needs to know. It does not attempt to cover the specific needs of people with various body and movement impairments. People with various chronic or acute physical problems may in fact need to adopt postures or ways of working that would be uncomfortable or inappropriate for people without such conditions. In addition, this book will not attempt to speak specifically about all the common variations in body build that can affect how people position themselves at their desks. For example, a woman with very large breasts will have extra weight pulling her shoulders forward as she sits and types. Or someone who is very overweight may not be able to sit as close to their desk as they should to reach their keyboard in the best way. In these and other cases, the basic principles of body use detailed in the book will still apply, and concerned individuals will be able to experiment with their workstations and find ways to work in comfort.

This book focuses on a crucial element of computer use that has not had nearly enough attention paid to it—how to use your body as you work at your computer—how to move, sit, or stand for greatest comfort. And you will find that just a bit of time invested in learning about this will make a tremendous difference in your ability to use your computer comfortably.

KEY POINTS

- Using a computer safely requires relaxation, postural balance, proper movement technique, good equipment, and proper workstation setup.
- Body awareness is the foundation for safe and comfortable computer use. You have to *feel* your own body to know how to sit and move and to know what equipment will work for you, how to set it up, and how to use it.
- Don't adapt yourself to the requirements of your work or your workstation. Adapt them to your requirements. Change things. Create safety and comfort for yourself.
- Everything is connected. Your mind, your body, your life, your work, and your workstation form a seamless whole. Pay attention, work patiently at change, pace yourself, and you will enjoy the process of change and succeed at it.

BODY AWARENESS IS THE KEY

A number of years ago, I taught a workshop on body awareness and workplace safety. At the end of the workshop, one of the executives who had attended shared an insight with the group. He related that his factory had a fairly high rate of back injuries but that the whole back-safety program had been discontinued because it simply didn't work. The employees were given all the right advice about body mechanics, but having the employees take the course didn't actually reduce the number of back injuries.

The insight the executive gained through his experiences at the workshop was simple, yet profound: the employees were told to lift with their legs, not their backs, but they didn't know in their own bodies exactly where their legs stopped and their backs began.

Intellectual information about your body isn't enough to help you avoid computer discomfort. You also have to learn to *feel* your body. Changing from strained movement and work habits to comfortable, safe patterns means being able to feel the different effects of different body movements, feel which movements are better, and then choose the better way of working.

By doing the experiments and practices described in this book, you will learn how to monitor your body and notice signs and sensations of tension and misuse. You will learn how to figure out what to do to correct the problems you detect. And you will learn what comfort really is.

BODY AWARENESS

What is body awareness? Being aware of your body means *consciously* noticing your body—feeling its position, its movement, its tone. This next experiment is an exercise I picked up many years ago from Timothy Gallwey's book *Inner Tennis*.

EXPERIMENT: RAISING ARM

What does it mean to pay attention to your body? How do you pay attention to your movements? How do you know when you are doing a good job of paying attention? This experiment will begin to answer these questions for you.

There are two parts to this experiment. *Don't read the second part before you do the first part.*

FIRST PART: Stand up in a comfortable position, with your arms down by your sides. Now, raise one arm up over your head. That sounds pretty simple, right? Try this before going on to read the second part.

SECOND PART: Standing up again, raise your arm over your head, to the same position—but this time pay careful attention to experiencing every detail and every inch of the process of raising your arm.

What differences did you feel in those two ways of raising your arm? Most people find the two movements very different. In the first, people generally are aware of where the arm started and where it finished, but they don't notice much about what goes on in the movement between the end points. They pay attention to the end points of the movement but not to the process of movement.

When they raise their arms the second way, most people slow down the movement a lot, and they pay attention to the feeling of the movement. This is what it means to pay attention to your body and yourself. It means to devote attention to *how* you move and *what* you feel. It means paying attention to the present moment and all the sensations in your body. It is not a matter of looking up and away, thinking *about* your body, distancing yourself from it and analyzing it. Paying attention to your body means focusing into your body in an ongoing, feeling, sensing way.

• • • • • • •

By the way, in many of the exercises in this book, I talk about what "most people feel." That is a way of focusing the discussion on the responses and experiences that I have seen in my teaching to be most common. That doesn't mean that different responses or experiences are wrong. You may feel something different, and that is fine.

If we were doing the exercises together, I could address the specific experiences you have, but in writing a book, I have to talk about what most people will usually feel. If you find yourself experiencing significantly different results in some exercise, that can be the starting point for heightened awareness of your particular movements and ways of being in your body.

Did you feel in this experiment what I suggested most people would feel? Did you feel something different? Did you feel nothing at all? Perhaps all that you felt was *confused*. Try not to let it worry you. Many people feel confused when they begin body awareness training. It's so new and different. Just keep on reading through the book and doing the exercises. If one exercise doesn't click for you, then another one will. As you get farther on in the book, it will make more and more sense to you. At that point, you might wish to go back to earlier exercises that didn't work for you and try them again. As your sensitivity to and understanding of your body and the exercises increases, you will probably understand exercises that were confusing the first time around.

• • • • • • •

Most of us go through our daily lives with our attention focused on goals and problems. We direct our attention outward at what we are trying to do or get, and by and large we ignore ourselves as we move and act. Have you ever just sat at your computer, working away, not noticing that your body was tense and uncomfortable in some minor, background way? Until the minor background annoyance got so painful that all of a sudden you did notice it? At that point, you may have been surprised by the sudden pain. However, if you had been paying attention all along, you would have noticed the small faint beginnings of discomfort and done something about it before it turned into a serious pain.

By learning how to pay attention to the *process* of working at a computer you will be nipping problems in the bud. Once you know how to pay attention to your body, you will find that it will take only a few seconds now and again to make the small adjustments necessary to ensure that you can use your computer in comfort. Of course, in addition to knowing *how* to pay attention, you will also have to know *what* to pay attention to, and most of the book will deal with that.

• • • • • • •

When you investigate your way of working at your computer, what things do you investigate? The first and most concrete thing to examine is sensations of strain in muscles and joints. What position are you in, and how do you hold yourself in that position?

Paying attention means feeling how tense or relaxed your muscles are, whether your breathing is relaxed and full, and whether your posture is balanced and easy or imbalanced and strained. Paying attention means feeling how all your muscles and movements affect one another.

Here comes an important idea:

Every part of your mind/body is connected to every other part of your mind/body. What you do in one part of your self influences what you do in your whole self. ("Mind/body" may seem like an odd term to you, but in the field of body awareness education it is a common term, which arose as an attempt to find one word for the whole human being.)

EXPERIMENT: TENSION

There is a very simple experiment which will help you feel this interconnectedness. Put a pencil down on the floor, and walk back about ten feet from it. Now walk over, pick it up, carry it over to a new spot about ten feet away, and put it back down. This is your normal way of moving. Nothing special.

Now, tighten up one shoulder. Each person will have their own way of understanding and doing that. You might scrunch your shoulder and pull it down. Someone else might brace their shoulder and push it up. Whatever you want to do is fine. While keeping your shoulder tight, pick up the pencil and move it back to the first spot.

Does keeping your shoulder tight change your overall movements? When you tighten your shoulder, do you tighten other parts of your body? Which parts? Most people notice that when they tighten one part of their body they tighten a lot of other parts as well.

Some people will notice very little even when there are major changes in their movement. Many people are so unused to examining or feeling their bodies that they simply miss much of the rich detail of their physical being. If you happen to be in that situation, don't give up. If you just keep on practicing, you will become more physically aware, and you will find that awareness more interesting and more helpful than you can possibly anticipate now.

Just to carry the idea to an extreme, scrunch up your nose as tight as you can, hold it that way, and walk around. Now let your nose loosen, and walk around again. Does tension in your nose affect your feet? Most people find that it does.

You can try the experiment again tightening other parts of your body. Does it make a difference which part you tighten? You could also try loosening a particular part of your body. Perhaps let one knee get too loose and wobbly. Or let one arm hang down limp. Does that also affect your overall way of moving?

Imagine sitting at your computer. Perhaps you hold your head cocked a bit to one side. When you do that, you tighten muscles on one side of your neck. And when you do *that*, you tighten other muscles throughout your body. Or perhaps you hold your shoulders too tight as you type. Will that create excess tension in your low back?

Sometimes the postural tension in people's bodies stems from old injuries. As a general rule, when we hurt ourselves, we automatically

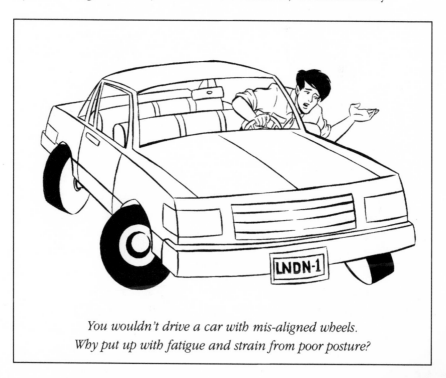

You wouldn't drive a car with mis-aligned wheels.
Why put up with fatigue and strain from poor posture?

stiffen up to restrict movement of the injured part and protect it from further injury and pain. However, by the time the injury is healed, the bracing has often turned into an unconscious postural habit, which will persist in a minimal way until something is deliberately done to eliminate it. Sometimes the injured part is simply weak and you are bracing it to withstand the stress of long hours at the computer. If you feel that old injuries are contributing to discomfort at your computer, you may wish to consult a professional to deal with that.

Everything is linked to everything else. Your body is like a web. If you pull on one strand, every strand gets tugged on. Learning how to *pay attention* to and *feel* the interconnections throughout the whole web is the beginning of being able to use a computer comfortably.

• • • • • • •

Not only can you pay attention to different parts of your body, but you can pay attention to what you think and feel and how that affects your body. Your mind and body are not really separate. They are just different elements of the same whole. What you think and feel directly affects your muscles and your posture.

EXPERIMENT: WANTING

Put a pencil on the floor, and then stand about ten feet away. Stand up comfortably. Look at the pencil. Oh, I forgot to tell you, this is a magic pencil. With this pencil you can write your own ticket. Really. Whatever you write with this pencil will come true. You could have a solid gold sports car or a swimming pool filled with chocolate ice cream. You get the idea. Wouldn't you love to go over and get that pencil?

Build up within yourself a feeling that this is really a wonderful pencil and you would really like to have it. Actually *intend* to go over and get the pencil. You have seen little kids visibly *wanting* to go pick something up to play with. It must be that kind of authentic wanting. You must feel it in your body.

It is important to be clear about what wanting the pencil means. "Wanting" is not the same as "going." Don't actually walk over and get the pencil. Focus instead on the *feeling* of wanting to go over.

It is also important not to become stiff and rigid. When I say not to actually move to go get the pencil, I don't mean that you have to make your body absolutely motionless. Don't freeze up and physically prevent your body from moving in order to focus on wanting to move. Just let your body experience the wanting and react to it naturally and spontaneously.

A third difficulty in this experiment is that "wanting" does not mean merely *thinking about* getting the pencil. There is a difference between "thinking about" loving someone and actually feeling love for them. *Thinking about* is more of a disconnected intellectual picture, but *feeling* is something you do with your "heart" and your body. Relax, be natural and create an authentic feeling in your mind/body of desire and intention to walk over and get the pencil. Most people can create this feeling when they focus on it, though many need some personal guidance to home in on it.

What happens when you stand and focus on wanting the pencil? Take some time to let the feeling build. Once you establish this feeling, you will probably feel yourself "involuntarily" tipping toward the pencil. For most people, this movement will be a small drift toward the pencil, perhaps an eighth of an inch (about a third of a centimeter) or so, though some people will actually move quite a bit. Most people will feel as though a magnet is gently drawing them toward the pencil. (Some people will actually tip away from the pencil or move in other directions, and those responses often have to do with whether they feel they are allowed to move toward what they want or have to pull away from it.)

The idea that thoughts immediately create body responses may be very new to many people. Some people believe so deeply that their minds and bodies are not connected that they cannot figure out how to build up the in their bodies the feeling of authentic wanting. Some people are so unused to paying attention to the experience of body processes that even when they actually move toward the pencil they do not notice it. A different way to think about this exercise may help you do it.

In the 1930's, Edmund Jacobson did a series of electromyography experiments involving muscular responses to imagery. He found that if he asked a person to imagine moving a body part, there were nerve impulses directed to precisely the muscles that would actually move the body part in an ordinary movement—even when there were no movements that were observable externally. In other words, there is scientific evidence for the idea that what you think, you do.

When you have an image of a movement and intend to execute the movement, your brain sends nerve impulses to the muscles that will do the movement. The muscles can act with a range of force, from a barely perceptible tensing to an all-out clenching. However, even below the range of what is barely perceptible to most people, there is still activity, the faintest stirrings of the muscles. You could call these faint, normally imperceptible tensings "micromovements."

The pencil-wanting experiment is a way to help you begin to notice the micromovements that are the small beginnings of the action of going to get the pencil. The experiment is an attempt to help you make the imperceptible perceptible. With training, you can sensitize yourself to events that are an ordinary part of human existence but which almost everyone ignores.

This experiment makes it quite clear that there is an intimate connection between your mind and body. All you have to do is wish to begin moving in some direction and your body will begin to perform that movement. That is not surprising when you think about it. The body is, after all, the way we go about doing what the mind wants. But feeling this, experiencing it, gives us a lived experience of the fact that there is no separation between the mind and the body, even though the structure of our language forces us to talk about them as separate, different things. (Of course, though there is no separation, we often wish to discuss specifically either the mental or the physical element of human experience, so having language that distinguishes between mind and body is useful.)

When you start to pay attention to where and how you focus your attention, you will start to feel your body much more clearly. You will probably discover that there are dull spots in your body, parts of your body that you don't normally feel or pay much attention to. However, the only way to make sure that you are using your body correctly as you work at the computer is to feel all of your body.

EXPERIMENT: FEELINGS

Paying attention to yourself includes noticing your feelings and how they affect your body and your movements.

Imagine that you have to write a report for someone who is always rude and demanding. He yells at you when he doesn't get what he wants, and he never bothers to thank you when you do give it to him. How do you feel? Irritated perhaps? Maybe resentful. Perhaps you really would rather chuck the report in the wastepaper basket. Get into these feelings of resentment. Let them build in you.

Notice what your body is doing when you are feeling these negative emotions. How do these emotions affect your breathing and muscle tension? How do they affect your posture? How do they affect the rhythm and quality of your movements? Most people will notice that anger and resentment increase their physical tension and restrict their breathing. The increased tension makes movements stiff and difficult, and strained movements create wear and tear on the body.

If you stagger along every day under the weight of a lot of emotional stress, that will affect the balance, ease and comfort of everything you do, including the physical act of typing on the computer keyboard. If you are anxious about using your computer, that will tense up your body, make using your computer even less comfortable, and make you more anxious about using it. Paying attention to yourself includes paying attention to your feelings and how they affect your body.

One caution about feelings and body use: sometimes the way people breathe or hold themselves is related to deep emotional wounds. For example, someone who was beaten a lot as a child may hold their shoulders hunched up as though waiting for another blow all the time. That posture would significantly increase the stress of using a keyboard. The body awareness training in this book may be only the beginning of what is necessary to help a person correct a postural problem that in reality is much more than a simple postural problem.

HOLISM

This book takes a holistic viewpoint. Every exercise affects all the others. Every part of your body affects every other part of your body. Your feelings affect your body and vice versa. The office environment affects your body, and how you act certainly is part of what shapes the office environment. Life is an interdependent web.

The three body awareness experiments you have just done demonstrate this interdependence. What you do affects how you perform. What you want affects how you perform. And what you feel affects how you perform. You need to pay attention to what you do, want, and feel as part of learning to work with computers in comfort.

The crucial element in learning to work in comfort is learning how to pay attention to *yourself* as you work at your computer. The more you notice, the more information you will have at your disposal in analyzing and correcting discomforts.

By learning to pay attention to your feelings of fatigue and strain, you will be able to identify and eliminate their causes. Learning to use computers comfortably will start with identifying and creating feelings of relaxation, freedom and ease. Once you experience those feelings, they will be your test and guide in working at your computer. Anything that takes you away from comfort and into the realm of stress and strain must be changed.

In order to keep your body as relaxed and balanced as possible, it is necessary to examine *all* the workplace stresses that affect you. The next chapter will examine the nature of computer stress.

RESOURCES

"Somatic education" is the umbrella term usually used to refer to the large variety of body/movement awareness disciplines. Each discipline takes a somewhat different approach to mind/body use, and all the disciplines have something to contribute to the broad picture.

The body awareness work that is the heart of *Comfort at Your Computer* is part of Being In Movement® mind/body training, the method that I have developed. For more information on this method, see Appendix C.

If you are interested in body awareness training in addition to what is included in this book, aside from contacting me about *Comfort at Your Computer* workshops and consultations (see Appendix A), you could look around your community for teachers of such disciplines as Aikido, yoga, the Feldenkrais Method® of somatic education, or the Alexander Technique. One way to get information about these and other body disciplines is through searching the World Wide Web.

For books and tapes about the Feldenkrais Method, or to find a Feldenkrais practitioner, you can contact the Feldenkrais Guild®, 524 Ellsworth Avenue SW, Albany, OR 97321 USA. Phone 800-775-2118. E-mail feldngld@peak.org, or visit http://www.feldenkrais.com. Another source for Feldenkrais books and audiotapes is: Feldenkrais Resources, 830 Bancroft Way #112, Berkeley, CA 94710, USA. Phone 800-765-1907. E-mail Feldenres@aol.com, or visit http://www.feldenkrais-resources.com.

Be aware, of course, that other practitioners will take different approaches to somatic training than shown in this book and may or may not have much experience with computer use.

For a very interesting map of the broad field of bodywork and somatics, see *Discovering the Body's Wisdom*, by Mirka Knaster, Bantam Books, 1996.

KEY POINTS

- You have to feel your body in order to know what you are doing and what to change. Practice becoming consciously aware of your body—noticing and feeling its position, its movement, its tone. Pay attention to the process of action, not just the goal.
- It is OK to feel confused as you begin working with body awareness. That is part of the process of exploring new, unmapped territory.
- Your movements, your desires, and your feelings affect every aspect of your whole mind/body. The more you notice about yourself, your workstation and your work, the more information you will have at your disposal in analyzing and correcting discomforts.

3

WHAT IS COMPUTER STRESS?

This book is about comfort. And it's also about the opposite of comfort—stress. Stress is what keeps you from being comfortable at your computer. So we have to ask an important question: What is computer stress?

EXPERIMENT: YOUR IDEA OF STRESS

Take a couple of minutes to think about the following questions. You may find that writing down your answers will help you organize your thoughts.

What do you think stress is?

What do you think computer stress is?

What discomforts do you experience when you work at your computer?

What are the sources of computer stress?

Do you think it is possible to work at your computer without feeling stress?

How would you do that?

WHAT IS STRESS?

The word *stress* is commonly used in three ways. It can refer to things which are challenging or threatening. It can refer to the physical and mental responses to a challenge, responses such as muscle tension, increased pulse rate, or feelings of anxiety. And the word can also refer to the physical and emotional damage that results from undergoing long-term stress responses. One way to make this distinction between challenges, responses, and results clearer is to use three different terms. The word *stressor* is often used to refer to any external object or event which is a challenge or threat. *Stress response* would then refer to the internal mind/body responses to stressors. And *stress-related illness* would refer to the conditions that can result from long-term stress.

Imagine that you're walking through the jungle. All of a sudden, a tiger springs out at you. The tiger is the particular stressor you have to deal with. And the pounding of your heart and the shaking of your legs are the fight-or-flight stress responses you experience in your body. In the ordinary way we use the word *stress*, the tiger would be a stress confronting you (the first sense of the word), and the shaking would be the stress you feel (the second sense of the word).

Imagine that the tiger jumps out at you a dozen times a day, day after day. You will be subjected to a constant, long-term challenge or stressor. You will also experience constant, long-term stress responses and might eventually wind up with physical or psychological problems from the wear and tear on your body/mind. These problems would be stress-related illnesses or injuries (the third sense of the word).

A tiger, however, is a simple example. If you are new to working with a computer, and your computer makes you anxious, is the computer a stressor? Well, yes, sort of. But it is a stressor only because you are stressed by it. The computer itself is just a hunk of metal, plastic and glass. It is not threatening in the way that a tiger really is threatening. The computer is a stressor because of the fears you bring to working with it.

Also, the stress you feel when you sit down to work at your new computer for the second time is to some extent a product of your memories of the stress you experienced the first time. If you are afraid that working at the computer will be stressful, then it probably will be. And if you keep working at the computer and keep being stressed out by that, eventually you will develop some stress-related illness, and that too will be stressful. So part of the stress that will make the illness worse will be the stress of having the illness. The point is that there isn't a clear separation between stressors, stress responses, and stress-related illnesses in our daily lives.

A chair that is too small for you really is a stressor. It puts strain on your body as you sit in it. If you have a good chair and sit in it with poor posture, you may find the chair uncomfortable, but the chair isn't really a stressor. It is what you bring to the chair that is the problem. Often we make situations stressful through our mental and physical habits. Though the words *stressor* and *stress* may be clearer and more specific, I think that the common, less specific use of the word *stress* is really more faithful to what our lives are like. In this book, I will often use the more general word *stress* and only occasionally use the more specific terms *stress* and *stressor*.

Your computer, your workstation, and your work environment as a whole can include many different stress factors. There may be external elements that are physically or emotionally stressful. *Physical stressors* may include such things as glare on your computer screen, a desk that forces you to adopt an awkward work position, or the requirement that you type at top speed for many hours every day. *Psychological stressors* may include such things as a rude and demanding boss or an impossible-to-meet deadline.

Some stress factors are not really part of the external work environment but are part of your physical, behavioral, or psychological makeup. If your back is weak because of a car accident a number of years ago, that physical condition may make sitting and typing painful. If you normally sit with your head cocked over to one side as you work, that postural habit will produce strain and pain. If you are an angry person, you may bring that with you to your work and get enraged at your computer when it crashes and loses data. Such emotional turmoil will produce a lot of wear and fatigue over the long run.

Postural strain factors are habitual ways of holding yourself and moving that are anatomically awkward and imbalanced and which can produce stress responses and stress-related injuries or illnesses. *Emotional strain factors* are habitual fearful and/or antagonistic ways of feeling and acting and which can produce stress responses and stress-related illnesses or injuries.

We could call such conditions predisposing stress factors. They aren't stressors, but they produce stress responses—when the matching environmental trigger is present. Holding your head cocked a bit to the side might not be a problem in your life—until you need to sit and type for hours on end. The idea that stressors are challenges and stress responses are what we do in response to the challenges is too simplistic. Very often challenges are challenges mostly because of how we respond to them. Very often the internal and external stress factors are all part of one another. And very often the stress responses are part of the challenge.

That is the reason that we ordinarily use just one word to refer to physical and psychological stressors, postural and emotional strain factors, and all the various emotional and physical stress responses and injuries. They are all wrapped up in each other. Emotional stresses result in physical discomfort, and physical stresses are emotionally draining. Postural and psychological stresses aggravate each other, and they often reflect each other.

The various stresses and stressors all affect and amplify one another. Stress factors add up. In fact, they multiply. The more stress you experience, the more bothered you will be by things that wouldn't ordinarily be too bad. If your back is already sore, then sitting at your desk typing for two hours may be very stressful. In this book, you will have the opportunity to pry apart the different kinds of stress and learn ways of handling each one.

GENERAL EFFECTS OF COMPUTER STRESS

Computer stress refers to discomfort caused by working at a computer. Working at a computer can cause a variety of mental and physical conditions. Many of these conditions are also effects of general life stresses, and so computer use may not really be separable from the rest of your life. In any case, if you find yourself recognizing any of these conditions in yourself, it is time to think about what you need to change in your life.

Spending hours in a fixed position typing can be very fatiguing. Overusing a body part creates localized wear and tear in muscles and surrounding tissues and nerves. There can be inflammation, pain, swelling, soreness, tingling and numbness. There can be pain and soreness in the neck, back, legs, arms, hands and fingers. There can be headaches and eye strain. There can be feelings of tightness and stiffness.

A term that you will hear often is *repetitive strain injuries* (RSI). This refers to injury, pain, or disability caused by a task that uses a body part over and over in the same way for long periods of time, especially while the body as a whole is held in a relatively stationary position.

Other common terms that mean the same thing are *repetitive motion injury* (RMI), *cumulative trauma disorder*, or *overuse syndrome*.

Beyond the localized wear and tear, computer stress can cause or contribute to conditions (which are often stress-related) such as insomnia, irritability, chronic fatigue, cardiovascular disease, gastrointestinal disease, alcoholism, and so on.

Of course, the effects of computer stress are not limited to the individual working on the computer. A stressed-out computer worker may well treat her or his co-workers, friends, and family badly. Somewhere there is a computer worker who has gone home swearing at his computer and kicked his dog in frustration.

Computer stress also affects the workplace. It creates tension and interpersonal friction, and it affects the financial health of the company by reducing the worker's concentration and output and increasing his or her on-the-job errors. In addition, computer stress results in direct medical and psychological treatment costs, and it results in the indirect costs of training replacement workers, higher insurance, litigation, and the time spent on all these factors.

Society as a whole also is damaged by computer stress. Large numbers of people are now spending considerable amounts of time working with computers, and if people must endure unsafe and unhealthful work environments, society pays through increased medical costs and social disruption.

IDENTIFYING STRESS

The most direct effects of computer stress are changes in your muscles, breathing, and posture. Learning to notice those physical changes will help you identify and change the stress conditions that affect you as you work at your computer.

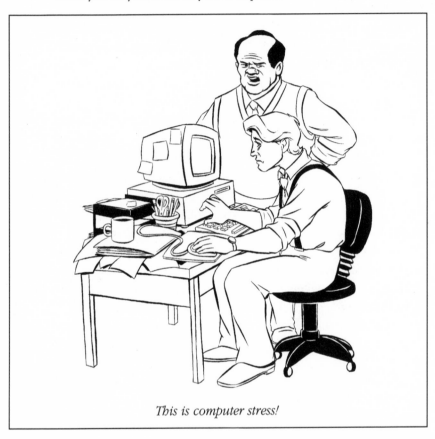

This is computer stress!

I'm sure you can recognize stress when you see it. How do you think the guy in the cartoon feels? He has physical stressors and emotional stressors piled on top of each other. Postural strain as well. And perhaps also the emotional strain of thinking that he can't do his work, that he'll never get a promotion, and that he's a loser.

EXPERIMENT: FEELING STRESS

Can you do more than merely imagine how the guy feels? Can you step into his shoes and actually feel in your own body what he must feel in his? What does his neck feel like? All his muscles must be tight as wires. What does his stomach feel like? Tight and churning. With his boss standing there beside him fuming, he probably feels like wrenching himself away and running or hiding. Or perhaps he is angry, swearing silently to himself, just about ready to punch his boss.

If you really enter into the feeling of the cartoon, you will actually feel stress responses in yourself. What do you feel happening in your body as you feel that stress?

What is happening to your breathing? Most people experience that their breathing gets shallow, rapid, and tight.

What is happening to your muscles? Do specific muscles get affected more than others? Do different muscles get affected differently? Do you move parts of your body? Most people experience that their muscles get tense. Very often people experience the greatest tension in their jaw, neck, shoulders, and belly, though of course many other areas may be tensed as well.

What is happening to your posture? Do you change the placement of specific areas of your body? Does your whole body change? Many people experience that they pull their heads down, hunch up their shoulders, and cave in their chests.

What happens to your attention? What do you pay attention to? Does your attention get broader or narrower? Most people experience that their attention becomes very narrow. They can't pay clear attention to much that is going on in and around them.

All these changes are the physical basis for the experience of stress. Notice that often we experience these changes as *happening* to us. In actual fact, these changes are *actions*, and we are *doing* these physical actions, though generally without awareness of our active role in the *doing*. Even though we may not be aware of doing stress, simply becoming aware of our stress responses is the first step in refraining from doing stress.

People often think of stress as something psychological or emotional, but fundamentally stress is physical. It is what happens in your body when you are confronted by stressful events and situations. If nothing out of the ordinary happened in your body—if your breathing remained calm, and your muscles remained relaxed, and your posture stayed balanced—then you wouldn't be doing/feeling any stress.

The muscular/postural essence of the stress response in the body is compression and imbalance, and this is what we will focus on in identifying and changing stress. When people experience stress, they compress and distort their muscles, breathing, posture, and movement. Distortion can be twisting, shrinking, puffing up, and so on—anything that distorts the posture. Compression most often takes the form of tense constriction, though it can also manifest as limp collapse. One person might tighten her shoulders and her neck. Another person might let his head hang down and his posture slump. Both people will experience pressure in their bodies, one from active muscle constriction and the other from weight hanging passively down.

MUSCULOSKELETAL ASPECTS OF COMPUTER STRESS

Understanding the musculoskeletal basis of stress is important in identifying and reducing computer stress.

MUSCLE ACTION: The first thing to understand about the muscles that move us around is what they do. (There are other kinds of muscle, such as the heart muscle, but this discussion focuses on the skeletal muscles.) Muscles are bundles of fibers. The fibers shorten when the nerves send them a message to do so. The percent of fibers told to shorten can vary, and it is this which produces variations in muscular effort. If all the fibers in a muscle are told to shorten, then the muscle is putting out its maximum effort.

Muscles do only one real, active movement: they shorten. When they shorten, they pull on the bones they are attached to, and this is what causes movement. Muscles shorten, and when they are told to stop, they cease to shorten. In other words, they stop working. They relax and get longer again. When a muscle ceases to shorten, it falls back to its uncontracted length. Note that muscles do not expand, they just give up contracting.

There are two problems people commonly experience that concern shortening of muscles. One is habitual tension, in which people have developed the habit of continuously shortening a muscle. The other problem is that many people, in their efforts to relax, use effort. That is, they do something active to pull on or shake loose their muscles. But any activity is more work, just the opposite of relaxation. (It is true that tensing one muscle can relax another. Muscles work in pairs around joints. One muscle bends the joint in one direction, and the opposite muscles pulls the joint in the opposite direction. Normally, a reflex acts to relax one muscle when the other muscle tenses. However, in chronic tension, both muscles tend to be activated. In that case, increasing the tension in one muscle won't effectively relax the other, and that is why I prefer to avoid using tension in the pursuit of relaxation.) The solution to the problem of muscular tension is to *learn* to notice the intention to shorten the muscle and then to *learn* to stop intending it. This will be a key idea in the sections on relaxation and movement breaks.

STATIC AND DYNAMIC ACTION: There are two kinds of work that muscles can do, static and dynamic actions. A dynamic action is a normal movement, one in which the involved body part moves through space. An example of this would be moving your fingers up and down to strike the keys of your keyboard.

A static action is one in which muscular effort is directed toward holding the body or some body part stationary in space (or holding some other object stationary in space). An example of this would be holding your torso in a sitting position for an hour while you are typing.

In a dynamic action, the muscles that produce the movement change lengths as the body part being moved swings through its range of movement. In a static action, the muscles involved bring the body part to its required position, and then they *hold their length the same* as long as they keep the body part in the same position.

This difference in muscle movement between dynamic and static actions is very important. When a muscle acts, it tenses, and this tension squeezes the blood vessels that pass through it. In a dynamic action, the muscles involved tense to produce a movement and then relax when the movement is over. This alternating squeezing and releasing of the muscle acts as a blood pump. When the muscle is squeezed, blood is forced out, and when the muscle relaxes, blood rushes back in. Because of this, a muscle doing hard work receives a good deal more blood than a resting muscle. This pumping action is what keeps the working muscle supplied with nutrients and oxygen. The pumping action also flushes away the waste products that the muscle produces as it works. In a dynamic action, the muscle is constantly fed and cleaned as it works.

EFFECTS OF STATIC ACTION: When a static action is performed, the muscles involved tense and then maintain that tension without varying it. The muscle squeezes without any letup, and blood is forced out of the muscle. There is no pumping action, and blood flow to the muscle is diminished, which reduces nutrition and cleansing of the muscle. When the muscle is exerting even as little as fifteen percent of its maximum strength in a static action, it is working so hard that the blood supply cannot keep up with the metabolic demands of the muscle. That means that the muscle begins to be starved for oxygen and nutrients and drowned in its own waste products.

Fatigue is the inability of the muscle to keep doing its work due to build-up of waste products. Dynamic work can lead to fatigue, of course, but static work is considerably more fatiguing simply because the waste products are not carried away and build up faster. If you rest when you feel the weakness and pain of fatigue, the muscle will recover. However, if you subject the muscle to static action and overuse every day over a long period of time, chronic fatigue builds up, and you will eventually damage the muscle. Damage can also occur to the ligaments, tendons, and joints associated with the muscles being used. This damage can include inflammation and degeneration.

Static action is also more wearing on the heart. In dynamic action, the heart rate rises to pump more blood to the muscles being used, but there is little change in blood pressure. In contrast, static action increases the blood pressure but there is not much increase in the pulse rate. Therefore in static action, the heart experiences greater strain than in dynamic action.

Static action also has an effect on the spinal column. The vertebrae are separated by cartilage disks. These disks do not have a blood supply, but instead are nourished and cleansed by the diffusion of interstitial fluid into and out of the disks. (Interstitial fluid is the fluid that is ever-present in the body, between and around all the cells and organs.) Moving the vertebral column changes the location and amount of pressure on the disks. The disks are squeezed and released, which aids in pumping fluid into and out of the disks. In static action, there is less movement and therefore less pumping of fluid, which decreases the oxygen and nourishment available to the disks and the removal of waste products.

Psychological tension also contributes to the physical process of static action. Psychological tension is not merely psychological, after all. Psychological tension involves muscular tension, as everyone knows who has ever experienced how anxiety gives rise to tension in the neck and shoulders. Psychological tension really creates static loading in the muscles, so a work situation that involves static action and is emotionally tense is really doubly stressful.

An important effect of fatigue (whether from static or dynamic action) can be thought of as robbing Peter to pay Paul. If the work task fatigues the muscles that do the movements involved, often people will shift their postures or movements to use new body parts and muscles. These muscles and joints, however, are often not the first-choice ones that are naturally designed for performing the task movements, and the new postures or movements may be awkward and inefficient. They may put undue strain on the newly recruited joints and muscles and allow strain and fatigue to build up in the newly recruited body parts as well.

ENTRAPMENT OF NERVES AND BLOOD VESSELS: In many areas of the body, nerves and blood vessels pass between muscles, bones, and ligaments and are vulnerable to being squeezed and damaged. If the body is held in awkward postures, nerves and blood vessels may get directly compressed between bones.

Muscles and other soft tissue can also squeeze nerves and blood vessels. Soft tissue can be irritated through overuse or through compression due to awkward posture. When soft tissue becomes irritated, it will swell and press on the nerves and blood vessels passing through it. Compression combined with movement can be especially bad, since it will often cause greater irritation and swelling of the soft tissue than compression or overuse alone. Other conditions that cause swelling, such as arthritis or pregnancy, can also lead to compression of nerves and blood vessels. Muscle tension and spasm can also compress blood vessels or nerves that pass through the muscle.

When nerves are compressed, transmission of nerve impulses is impaired, and if the nerves are compressed over a long period of time, they may become damaged. Without proper nerve impulses to stimulate them, muscles become non-functional and can waste away. When blood vessels are compressed, blood supply to the body parts served by the blood vessels is reduced, and nourishment and cleansing of those parts is impaired.

CARPAL TUNNEL SYNDROME: There are a number of specific entrapment syndromes in which different areas of the body are affected in different ways. If you want more information about them, there are many books on work-related medical conditions.

Carpal tunnel syndrome is a common entrapment syndrome and one that many people have heard about. Carpal tunnel syndrome is so named because the small carpal bones in the wrist do form a tunnel. Actually, it is not so much a tunnel as an open ditch. The ditch, however, is covered by a ligament, so there really is an enclosed space, like a tunnel. Through that tunnel pass tendons for the muscles that move the fingers as well as the nerve that provides sensation for the thumb, the index, and middle fingers, and much of the palm. But the tunnel is small, and there is no spare room. If anything within the tunnel swells or if there is a reduction of the tunnel's width, the nerves and tendons that pass through the tunnel will experience friction and irritation.

If people spend long periods of time typing, the tendons that move the fingers and pass through the carpal tunnel can get irritated and swell, which in effect reduces the space in the tunnel and leads to more irritation. If the wrist is held bent backwards (hyperextended), that compresses the underside of the wrist and increases the pressure in the carpal tunnel. Unfortunately, many keyboards encourage this position, and many people type in this position even when keyboards don't require it. If the wrist is rested on the desk as a person types, that pressure also compresses the carpal tunnel. The swelling that is common in pregnancy can also result in compression in the carpal tunnel.

The impingement on the nerve and tendons in the carpal tunnel produces pain and weakness in the hand, wrist, and forearm, as well as numbness and tingling in the first three fingers, often first noticed at night. There may be clumsiness and restriction of movement. This is a serious condition that requires prompt medical treatment. (For information on the proper use of the hands in keyboarding, see Chapter 7.)

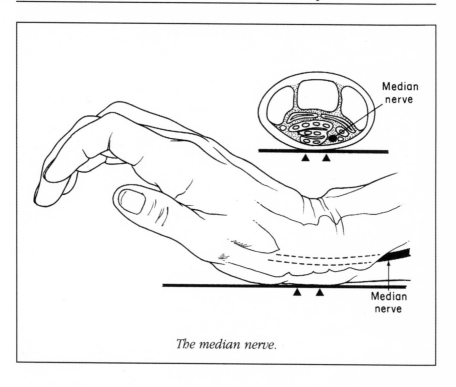

The median nerve.

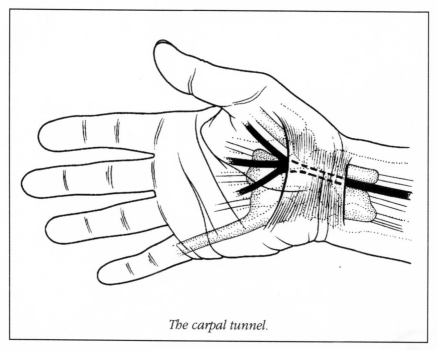

The carpal tunnel.

CAUSES OF STRESS IN COMPUTER WORK

Computer stress is not simple. Computer stress isn't caused by just one simple stressor. It has many causes, all of which interact and affect each other. Some of the sources of computer stress are personal, physical, emotional or social habits. Some of the sources of computer stress are part of the job design, the workstation setup or the work environment. Some of the sources are part of the interpersonal atmosphere of your workplace or the company philosophy and policies. And some sources are part of our society's values and culture.

There are many causes of computer stress that do not seem to be directly related to computer work at first sight. For example, though most people would not identify interpersonal friction as part of the problem of computer stress, it does affect how you feel and move. It would be very difficult for you to relax your body at your keyboard if the atmosphere in your office were tense and antagonistic. So getting along with your co-workers is in fact part of keeping your body relaxed and safe at the computer. In the same way, many other stress factors affect computer use, and a holistic approach is necessary for solving the problem of computer stress.

It is often hard to get a clear understanding of job-related stress simply because so many stress elements in our lives interact. You can think of yourself as a barrel and stress as water. You can hold only just so much water. If the only source of water in your life is your job, then a pretty wet job may be tolerable. However, if water is pouring in from family, financial, and health worries, and so on, then the water from your job may be the last bit that will fill the barrel to overflowing. At that point, you will not be able to handle the job, but it won't be just the job itself that you can't handle. And you will have to look beyond just the job in finding solutions that will let you handle your job well.

It will help you to be as aware as possible of all of the sources of computer stress. As you read through the following introductory survey of computer stress factors, think about whether any of them are present in your work. If some are present, notice your body's responses to those factors as you work. That will give you specific information about how stressful the stressor is and what you need to change and how. You can decide which sources are most important in your particular case, work on changing those that can be changed, and work on coping with those that cannot be changed.

Stressors are not absolute. How long and how intensely you are exposed to them can make them more or less stressful. The more time you spend at the keyboard, the greater the stress you will experience. Some things that are tolerable for a short time are intolerable for longer periods. In addition, some stressors that are overwhelming for one person, may be tolerable, harmless or even enjoyable for another person. Some people love mountain climbing and others are afraid of heights. In examining stress, you have to look both at your job and your ability to handle each different source of stress you face.

• • • • • • •

We can organize the specific stresses of computer work into a brief list. Which stress factors you experience will depend a great deal on the specifics of your work situation and your life. If you are working in a home office as a self-employed graphic artist, you will be in a very different situation than someone who is a data-entry clerk in a section of a department of a large company. As you read through the list, notice which stress factors stand out for you as part of your life or work.

POSTURE

One of the key factors in computer stress is strained, awkward posture. Some jobs by their very nature put people into awkward positions. Painting a ceiling, for example, forces you to bend your head back to look up. Sitting on a chair typing at a computer isn't quite that bad, but sitting is a very stressful task. Even worse, many people bring to that task poor habits of posture and body use that get them into trouble. We will go into this in great detail later in the book, but as just one example, I once worked with someone who came to me for movement lessons because he experienced low back pain when he typed. As I watched him, I immediately saw that he had a habit of cocking his head to one side, and it was that lopsided posture that stressed his back. He had never noticed that, and getting his head straight went a long way toward solving his problem.

Any position will wind up being stressful if you hold it long enough. And depending on how you set up your chair and workstation and the things you work with, you may force yourself to use more or less awkward postures.

MENTAL HEALTH

Being depressed, anxious or fatigued can certainly influence how you feel about your work and how you feel when you work. Your feelings aren't turned off when you turn on your computer. If you have had a death in the family, or have recently been divorced or have experienced some other major life event, that will have an effect on your ability to work in comfort.

Your emotional habits are important as well. For example, if you customarily feel angry and defeated when things go wrong, that will influence your work at your computer. Having deadlines, having your computer crash, having an electrical surge that destroys your hard disk—all these pressures and more are part of using computers. What you bring to your computer affects how you handle the pressures of work. Negative emotional habits will have a negative effect on concentration, productivity, and job satisfaction.

PHYSICAL HEALTH

If you are sick or have been injured, of course you will feel uncomfortable and have less energy. Working at your computer will demand a larger percentage of what you have to give. If the illness has been brought on by computer work, then the stress of computer work will feed on itself and grow. Imagine the stress of having to work at a computer even while it hurts, simply because the alternative is being unemployed.

Lifestyle factors are very important in determining how much energy you have and how good you feel. Drinking, smoking, not exercising, eating poorly, and not getting enough sleep will all make you feel drained and uncomfortable.

WORKSTATION

The way you set up your workstation is a crucial factor in creating computer stress. If you choose a poor chair, or set up your desk and computer wrong, you can place yourself in positions of torture. In the next section we will go into some detail about the musculoskeletal effects of poor working conditions, but for now it is enough to say that maintaining awkward postures for hours on end, repeating the same movements over and over, will cause damage to the body.

Later in the book, we will examine how you use your body and the relation this has to how you set up your workstation. There are a number of things to think about. How much physical pressure does your body exert on workstation surfaces—the floor, the chair, the desk, and the keyboard? What body parts take your weight, the softness or hardness of the support surfaces, whether your weight rests on rounded or sharp edge—all these elements affect your comfort. Friction with surfaces can be important, for example, in moving a mouse around your desk. And the amount of time you have to spend in contact with the surfaces is also important. Spending a lot of time with a major portion of your body weight resting on hard, rough, sharp edges will clearly be uncomfortable and damaging.

JOB DESIGN

Using a computer is not simply using a computer. For example, consider driving a car. Driving a car embraces a multitude of cars and drivings. I've never driven a high-powered race car around a track, but I'm sure it must be very different from driving my family minivan around town. Driving a car pulling a trailer is different from driving a car full of kids, and driving to the corner grocery store is different from rush-hour commuting or driving from Ohio to Oregon.

In the same way, the stresses you encounter in using a computer depend to a great extent on what you are using it for and how you are using it. What tasks are part of your job? What movements are part of the tasks? At what pace does your job demand that you work?

KINDS OF COMPUTER WORK: There are different kinds of computer work, and each kind puts different amounts of stress on different parts of the body. One kind of work is writing text, such as writing a novel, and this kind of work involves simple typing while keeping your eyes primarily on the screen. A second kind of work involves entering data from paper-source documents, and this work requires periods of uninterrupted keying, with your eyes primarily on the papers. If your data are primarily numbers, you would be typing primarily with one hand on the numeric keypad. A third type of work involves getting information from the screen, perhaps giving that information to people over the phone, and having your visual focus primarily on the screen. This kind of typing would not involve long periods of repetitive motion.

A fourth type of work involves a back-and-forth between the screen and paper documents or a person. This could be work in which you are receiving information and typing it into a computer document, or it could involve getting information from the computer and writing onto paper documents or telling it to a person. Rather than doing the same movements over and over for hours on end, in this kind of work you would experience much more variation of movement.

If your work involves interaction with people, are you talking to them over the phone? If so, do you use a regular telephone handset or a headset? If you use a regular hand-held telephone, you will be holding a telephone up next to your ear with one hand for long periods. Even worse, you may cock your head over and raise your shoulder to hold the telephone to your ear as you use both hands for typing. That tense, asymmetrical posture will be very stressful.

A fifth type of computer work is design and graphics work, and this could be anything from page layout, to engineering-design work, to generating computer art. The tasks are much less repetitive than simple data entry, and the movements involved may be less repetitive and monotonous.

A sixth use of the computer—though it may not be a form of work—is game playing. It may require a joystick or other extra input device, and it may require specific, very repetitive movements. Game playing may also involve high levels of excitement and tension.

DATA MANIPULATION: Does your job have rigid data manipulation formats that have to be adhered to? This kind of rigid detail work can be psychologically stressful. Does your job require a rapid pace of work and demand constant rapid finger movement? Does your job include constant monitoring of your pace? Aside from the high physical stress constant rapid movement entails, a forced-march pace of work with constant scrutiny is psychologically stressful. Jobs that force a human being to keep up with a fast-paced machine are very stressful. Jobs that allow workers to pace themselves or that naturally contain work pauses and variations in the work rhythm are much less stressful.

MOVEMENT REQUIREMENTS: It is important to consider what activities various parts of the body are required to do, either as primary movers or as supports for the primary movers. Does your work involve primarily simple typing movements, using one or both hands? Does your work involve the movements required in using a mouse or other non-keyboard input device? Does your work involve a lot of reaching movements, perhaps to get paper documents or turn pages? In these different tasks, your arms, shoulders, and back do somewhat different movements. It will be important to consider where the objects are placed that you must move and what their dimensions and weights are. Whatever the nature of the hand and arm movements in your particular computer task, does the rest of your body move? If not, then there is a constant muscular exertion to keep the body in place as a support for the arms, and that will be strenuous over the long haul.

If your whole body does move, what are the movements? Does the job require getting up and going places rather than sitting at the desk all the time? That would be much less stressful than maintaining a single constant posture. Does your job design require you to twist around toward just one side? Twisting or imbalanced movements done on a long term-basis are very stressful for the body.

REST BREAKS: Does your work have built into it opportunities for changing tasks and movements? Not being able to change tasks will increase boredom, as well as fatigue and strain. Does your job also include pauses for rest breaks? Are you able to pace your rest breaks and movement breaks according to your own needs? The time you spend in resting will more than be made up for by the improvement of task performance. Instead of working until you are so fatigued that you cannot work at all and then taking a rest, it is more efficient to use frequent rest breaks to prevent the onset of fatigue and performance degradation.

JOB DEMANDS: Jobs that demand too much or too little of the worker are also stressful. If there is too much responsibility for a given individual to handle, then the job will be stressful for him or her. If the worker has not been given adequate training and is not comfortable with the demands of the job, that will be stressful. If the work is too complex and hard to manage, it will also be stressful.

On the other hand, if a job involves repeating the same simple task over and over again, it will be monotonous and boring, and boredom itself is stressful to people. In addition, boredom leads to lethargy and decreased alertness, which increase errors and decrease productivity. Of course, there are individuals who find simple, repetitive work quite comfortable and are not bored by it.

People who do interesting and creative work with computers may be more engaged in the work, much less bored, and much less psychologically stressed by the work. Of course, this is the kind of work that requires much more varied movements and work pacing, so the work is less physically stressful as well, though it may include the stresses of deadlines, responsibilities, and difficult-to-solve problems.

SOCIAL INTERACTION: Another element to consider in the stresses involved in job design is social contact. Some people may find jobs that are socially isolated more boring and more stressful. Jobs that include interaction with other people may be more interesting, and there may be social support in dealing with the frustrations and stresses inherent in working. On the other hand, some people like solitude and some social interactions can be very stressful.

HOURS: And finally, the time of day is important. Working on a night shift is stressful since it disturbs the body's rest and sleep rhythms. Late in the work shift, a worker will be less rested than at the beginning of the shift. If a person is fatigued, she or he will have a harder time staying alert and will be more prone to errors.

PHYSICAL WORK ENVIRONMENT
The physical environment in which you work is also important. If the environment is cluttered, dirty, or cramped, that will affect how you feel. The quality of the indoor air and the temperature of the workplace also affect people.

Noise is important. Loud noises are stressful, and constant noise from computer fans, hard drives, dot matrix printers, and so on can add up as well. Conversation can be very distracting. Even more than handling just the noise of voices, trying to concentrate and not listen to the meaning of someone's words is stressful.

Lighting is important. There must be enough light to do the job well, but the lighting must not create glare or reflections on the computer screen.

INTERPERSONAL WORK ENVIRONMENT
The interpersonal environment at work also affects people. If your supervisor is demanding, rude, inconsistent, and blaming, that would certainly create a lot of stress. *Work* cannot be divorced from *human interaction*. People have to be treated decently to feel comfortable and work well. For purely financial reasons (if nothing else), it is important

for people in the workplace to learn and grow as human beings. We can all become more kind, tolerant, assertive, expressive, and cooperative, and that will help us function more productively in the workplace.

Role conflicts are stressful. If you have to answer to many different supervisors, that can create unclear job demands and be quite stressful. Privacy and overcrowding are other issues. Feeling exposed and not having a secure sense of spatial safety can be quite stressful.

Not being valued as an individual is stressful. Being treated unfairly or with prejudice is a major stress for employees exposed to such behavior. And treating others unfairly is also stressful. People who hurt others experience physical stress responses themselves from engaging in negative human interactions.

SCHOOL SETTING

Children are spending more and more time using computers for school work, and that is in addition to the time they spend playing computer and video games. It is important to make sure that they do not hurt themselves. Many children start off playing computer games when they are two or three years old. Imagine a twelve-year-old child who has been using computers for eight years. Imagine a twenty-two-year old who has been using computers intensively for eighteen years. They are at risk of developing incapacitating carpal tunnel syndrome or other computer-related injuries.

It is up to parents, teachers and school administrators to educate themselves about computer comfort and safety. When students are taught to use computers, they should be instructed in safety and injury prevention at the same time. Is this awareness part of the mindset of the school? Is care taken in computer labs and classes to ensure that the equipment fits the children and that they sit in relaxed, balanced ways? Are the students taught how to set up a workstation to minimize physical strain? Are they taught about appropriate movement breaks, and are they reminded to actually take breaks? Or are children working at adult-sized desks and tables simply because that's what is available? Are the students tense with effort or excitement? Do they get so engrossed in the computer work that they neglect to breathe or move?

Developing computer comfort and safety is crucial and, actually, quite simple, but it does take specific instruction. It takes interest and concern on the part of parents and teachers. However, it does not have to take a lot of time or money. Brief instruction in work safety can be included along with other computer instruction, and simple, inexpensive aids such as pillows and footrests can serve to adjust workstations to fit students.

COMPANY CULTURE

What values does your company culture hold? Does the company care about its workers? Or does the company consider workers to be replaceable units, worth less than the computers they minister to? If you don't feel that the company cares about your well-being, that will lead to resentment, dissatisfaction, absenteeism, and poor work performance. Not feeling respected is stressful.

Does the company care enough about workers to design jobs to minimize worker stress? For example, are jobs designed to incorporate rest breaks into the work? Are adjustable workstations provided so that people can fit the workstations to their physical requirements? Does the company train people in how to make the adjustments? Does the company provide a program of body awareness and ergonomics so that workers will know how best to set up and use their computers?

Work that promotes autonomy, responsibility, and creative use of an individual's talents is more satisfying to most people. Giving people a sense of control over their lives and a feeling that their creative energies are valued does a lot to create a positive work experience. Does your company value this kind of work atmosphere or not?

Work that includes social interaction and social support is generally a more positive experience. Does your company build opportunities for social interaction into the work? Does your company respond quickly and supportively to people's concerns about health and safety issues? Or does your company put itself in the position of an adversary, thereby adding stress to already stressful situations?

Does your company make efforts to ensure job security? Lack of job security can be very stressful, though some aspects of this may relate to the business performance of a whole industry, or the whole country, and be beyond your company's ability to control.

Does your company care enough to provide training in relaxation, communication and conflict resolution as part of the process of changing the workplace and relieving computer stress?

Of course there are many elements involved in your company's culture and way of treating workers. These questions should be just the starting place for thinking about this topic.

SOCIETY

Various social factors influence the amount of stress you feel at your keyboard. What values operate to convince us to maintain one posture or another as socially appropriate? What social values support or interfere with job satisfaction? What social values create or minimize stress?

One simple example of how social values affect the workplace stress, and thereby affect the physical stress you feel at your keyboard, is our society's devaluing of certain groups. If some people are paid less than others for the same work, or if certain groups are encouraged not to make full use of their talents, how does that make members of those groups feel about their jobs? How does that underlying current of dissatisfaction impact on *everyone's* experience of the workplace? Remember the exercises in Chapter 2 that helped you experience how your feelings and intentions immediately express themselves physically? You will notice other people's stress, even if only subliminally, and their stress will infiltrate your mind/body and cause you to feel stress as well. The stressful atmosphere caused by negative social values will translate into physical tension that will affect your wrists as you type.

We are all subjected to millions of messages from society about who we should be, how we should act, and what is valuable. Ideally society should deliver appropriate and respectful messages about what bodily beauty is, how we should use our bodies, how and how much we should work, and so on. These messages form the context of our self-image and our ways of working, and social influences must be taken into account in improving the ways we work at our computers.

Clearly it will be less than simple to engineer major changes in the interpersonal work environment, in the company culture and in society as a whole, as part of the task of reducing computer stress. However, it is interesting to think about this, and changes will come, even if slowly.

MAINTAINING COMFORT INSTEAD

Computer stress is not imaginary. It is not all in your head or something that can be triumphed over through sheer will power.

Computer stress is real. People who spend long hours working at a computer are running into the real physiological limits of the human organism, and those limits must be respected.

Stress is the result of having to face performance demands that are near or beyond the limits of the individual's abilities. It is important to remember that different people have different limits. One person is physically strong and flexible and finds sitting for hours at a computer no particular problem, while another finds long periods of sitting very painful. It is important to respect the reality of each person's limits. However, for all our differences, we are much the same, and there are some basic human performance limits. Spending a long time in an awkward posture maintained by static holding while doing a repetitive movement will be stressful for anyone.

Once you learn how to notice the causes of computer stress, you can take steps to deal with them. There are three interrelated steps that need to be addressed in achieving computer comfort. The first is reducing current levels of stress in your body. The second is the achievement of a positive mind/body state of openness, balance, power and ease. And the third step is reducing or eliminating external, environmental causes of stress.

Person, job, and society—all three areas are inevitably part of any work situation and all three can be improved. You can learn to use your mind/body as efficiently and economically as possible. Your job can be changed to bring it into accord with the design of the human being. And society can be changed so that the values we are taught are more humane.

Which should you try to change? Some companies prefer changing the worker so that the companies don't have to spend time and money changing their equipment and job designs. Some people would rather not have to take responsibility for how they live and move, and they would prefer that the company change. In reality, of course, both areas of change should be pursued. It will do little good to move gracefully and efficiently while you are subjected to intolerable working conditions. And it will do little good to provide excellent working conditions to people who misuse their bodies as they work and don't care to change. Working for social change is also important, though the immediate changes in the person and job are the easiest to implement and the most immediately effective.

KEY POINTS

- The word stress is commonly used to refer to three interconnected elements. It can refer to things that are threatening or challenging. It can refer to the immediate physical and mental responses to a threat. And it can refer to the physical and emotional damage that results from maintaining stress responses over a long period of time.
- Some stresses are the result of external emotional or physical pressures, and some stresses come from our own mental and physical habits. The various stresses all affect and amplify one another.
- The most direct effects of computer stress are constriction, collapse, and imbalance in muscles, breathing, posture, and movement. Pay attention to these physical changes. Use this awareness to identify and change the stress responses and the external conditions that affect you as you work at your computer.
- A dynamic action is a normal movement, one in which a body part is moved through space. A static action is one in which muscular effort is directed toward holding the body, some body part, or some other object, stationary in space. Long-term static actions are fatiguing and damaging to the body. Spending long periods repeating the same movements will also fatigue and damage the body. Keep moving and vary your movements!
- Many elements contribute to computer stress—everything from job design and workstation setup to postural and psychological habits, lifestyle and health, and social values. For greater comfort at the computer, reduce stress wherever you can.

SOFTENING
YOUR BREATHING

Compression is a fundamental element of the stress response, and the key to reducing stress is detecting and releasing compression in your body. You have to start by noticing the *sensations* of compression. Compression generally involves tension, tightness, and stiffness in muscles, breathing, posture, and movement. Paradoxically, compression can also stem from limpness. If you don't hold your body weight up, various parts of your body will hang down and cause pressure on other parts.

Releasing tension is the *undoing* part of overcoming compression. Finding a state of energized support is the *doing* part. The two themes of releasing and supporting will carry through all the body awareness exercises in *Comfort at Your Computer*.

• • • • • • •

Releasing the tension in your breathing is a good place to begin the process of stress reduction, and the best place to start softening your breathing is with developing an awareness of the core of your body.

Many people hold their pelvic musculature and bellies tense and sucked in. This produces a feeling of physical and emotional tension and constraint, though it may be so normal and familiar that it is never noticed. Have you ever been told to suck in your gut? That's anatomically unreasonable, though it seems to be a cultural imperative.

PRACTICE: RELAXING YOUR BELLY

Get up for a moment and walk around. What does your belly feel like? Do you suck your gut in? If you do, how does that affect your breathing?

How do you feel about your belly? Many people are ashamed of their bellies and try to hide them or make them look smaller.

In order to increase your awareness of how you hold the core of your body, consciously tighten your belly, anal sphincter muscles and genitals and then walk around. Really grip those muscles hard. Notice how stiff and strained this makes your legs, hips, and lower back and your movement as a whole. Notice how restricted it makes your breathing.

By the way, as you try this exercise, notice whether your clothes are comfortably loose. If they are tight, there will be a constant pressure on your body. Your muscles will actually tense up and fight the pressure, whether you notice it or not, and it will be hard to relax your belly. As a general rule, in relaxation and in everything else that will be discussed in this book, it will help to wear clothes that are as comfortable as possible.

Now, stand and alternate tightening your belly and relaxing it. Let it plop out when you relax it. Next try releasing your belly without doing a preliminary tightening. Along with softening your belly, for greater relaxation, consciously allow your genital and anal muscles to relax. Most people experience a noticeable release even when they had not first tightened their bellies consciously, and they realize from this that they had been unconsciously holding themselves tight and probably hold themselves tight all the time.

Try walking around again with your belly soft. How does that feel? Most people experience greater ease, fluidity, and solidity in their walk. And that is how walking should be—not tense and constricted. (Occasionally, people who are very stiff will experience discomfort when they relax their abdominal muscles. That is generally because they haven't relaxed and balanced the rest of their body when they relaxed their bellies.)

Holding tension in any area of your body makes all of your body uncomfortable, but the muscles in the belly, anus and genitals are especially important. They are the core of the body and the center of movement and balance. Holding tension in these body areas while sitting at the computer makes it impossible to relax, move freely, and work comfortably.

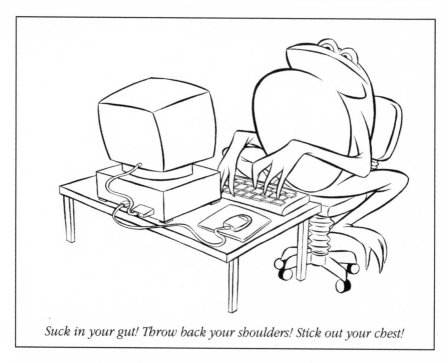

Suck in your gut! Throw back your shoulders! Stick out your chest!

Right about now you might be getting a little worried. Am I really recommending letting your belly stay relaxed? Yes, I am. I know that for many people talking about the body or feeling it is uncomfortable. We have been taught that the body is somehow "bad." Even worse is talking about the pelvis or the belly. However, using this whole area of the body properly is crucial in avoiding computer stress and creating computer comfort. If talking about this area of the body makes you uncomfortable, that emotional discomfort will translate directly into physical tension in the muscles of your pelvis and belly, which will interfere with your ability to sit comfortably at your computer. What we are doing here is just learning about the basic anatomy and engineering of the body. If you want the machine to run right, you have to learn about its construction and use.

Many people find the whole idea of letting their bellies relax totally unacceptable. Our culture has very specific ideas about how the body should be used and what makes a person nice to look at, and relaxing the belly is just *not* the thing to do! But let's take a look at some drawings. They are drawings of figures from advertisements that appeared in various places. Looking at ads is a good way of examining our culture's values. I find that the way advertisements show the body exemplifies our culture's ideals of strength and beauty, and I suspect advertisements go a long way toward shaping our ideals as well. Ads are effective when they tap into our ideals, and they also offer role models which shape them.

Drawing #1 was copied from a cookie wrapper and is a good illustration of the way we think about the body. When I show this to people in workshops, the overwhelming majority agree that the "correct" figure does indeed look much better than the "bad" figure. However, when I ask which man could more easily dodge a car that was heading right for him, almost everyone will choose the "bad" figure. People

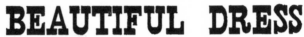

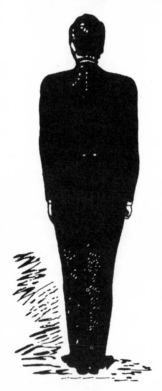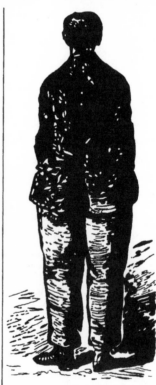

Proportions Correct.   Proportions Bad.

From a cookie wrapper.

easily recognize that the so-called bad figure is more relaxed, balanced and ready to move, but they have learned to believe that the tense, constricted, top-heavy, immobile figure is *good*.

This identification of beauty and power with tension can be seen in Drawing #2 as well. There is obvious tension in the face, the cock of the hips, and the wide stance. The text that went with the photograph was: "For the coolest guys only, tough new urban hardwear: just what you need to carry off a confident attitude." The verbal message reinforces the equivalence of power and tension by defining "cool" and "confident" as "tough" and stemming from hardness. There is an air of angry sexuality about the ad. The irony is that the man's stance is tense and immobile, just what would prevent him from moving easily and powerfully if he did have to fight off or escape from some attack. In particu-

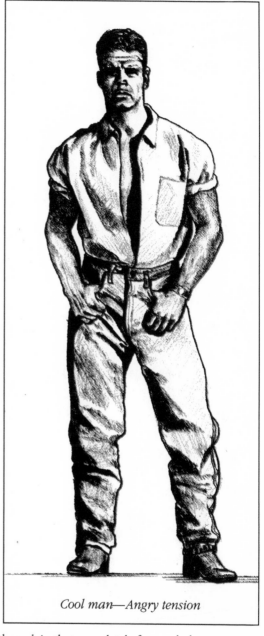

Cool man—Angry tension

lar, there is so much tension in the pelvis, that completely free and pleasurable movement there would probably be impossible too.

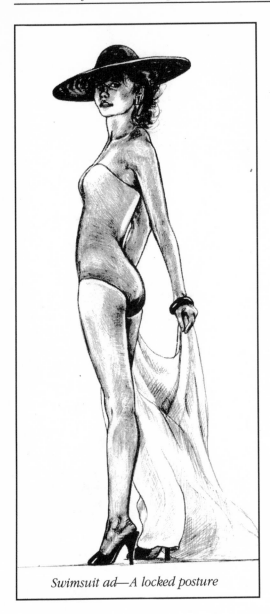

Swimsuit ad—A locked posture

Women, too, have their stylized ways of doing tension. Look at Drawing #3. This ad asks "What makes a swimsuit sexy?" And the answer is "Lots of beautiful shape." However, look at what is passed off as beautiful shape. Standing on high heels, the woman's feet are not in contact with the ground. Her knees, hips and low back are locked and rigid. Her left arm is held back in an awkward and tense position. (Try standing that way and see how you feel.) Her neck and face are tense. She is bound and rigid, without the softness that would allow her to move in the supple, balanced way that is the basis of grace and power. And yet when I show this photograph in workshops, people initially perceive the model as looking beautiful. Perhaps I am unusual, but I enjoy looking at people who are free, relaxed, powerful and graceful. I don't find tension, awkwardness and weakness beautiful.

Many ads showing women equate tension with beauty and strength, much as the men's ads do. There is, however, a second category of women's poses, and that is, for lack of a better term, the sex kitten pose. In this pose, women hold odd twisted positions, intertwining messages of helplessness and seductiveness. Again, most

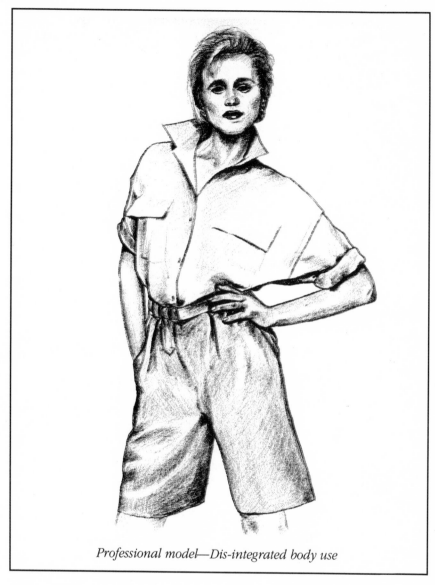

Professional model—Dis-integrated body use

people I show Drawing #4 to see the woman as beautiful and seductive. My first thought when I saw this photo was that the woman either had been in a serious accident or was a professional model. Notice how the head, shoulders and hips are cocked and twisted into angles in which the body is dis-integrated, broken into unrelated and uncoordinated pieces.

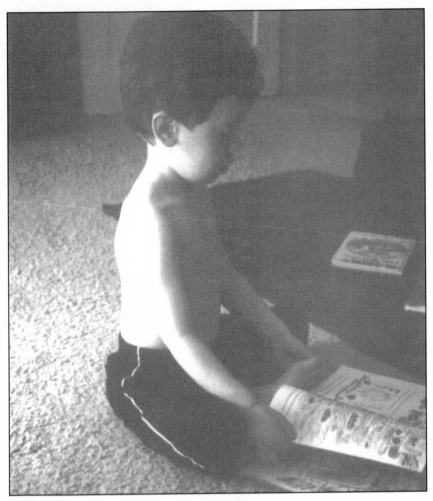

A postural ideal.

Just for comparison, examine Illustration #5, a photograph of my son I took when he was about four years old. Notice how effortlessly straight he holds his body. Rather than slumping over to look at the book he is reading, he rotates his head on top of his spinal column, maintaining efficient weight support while aiming his eyes downward. Notice that his shoulders are relaxed and rounded, his chest soft and his belly released. This is very close to what the cookie wrapper defined as "proportions bad," yet it is supple, graceful, strong, and balanced. When I grow up, I want to be as balanced and free as my son.

Our culture places trimness before us as the ideal of beauty, but if you look under the skin of that idea, *trimness* turns out to be another name for *tension*. Certainly exercising and being in good shape are good for you and are part of looking good. If you exercise and are in good shape, your belly and all the rest of you will be well-toned. However, the artificial trimness of postural tension and deliberate sucking in of the gut is *not* the same as being well-toned, and it is not good for you.

Sucking in your gut creates tension throughout the body. If you bring that dedication to tension with you to the computer, you are sitting down with two strikes already against you. In order to learn to work in comfort, you need to feel how your body operates and do what will make you truly relaxed and comfortable.

Almost always when I teach about relaxing the belly and letting it plop out I must spend time combating the notion that sucking in the guts looks better. People very quickly feel for themselves that they breathe and move more easily when they let their bellies out, but often they feel fat and sloppy. They feel embarrassed to go out in public looking relaxed and balanced. For many people it takes a good deal of practice to feel comfortable with being comfortable.

• • • • • • •

When I teach about relaxation, a question that always comes up is about the difference between relaxation and limpness. Relaxation is not just limpness, though many people think of it that way. I would

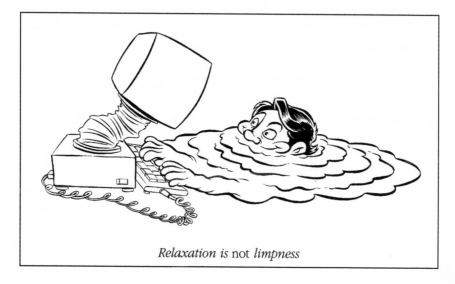

Relaxation is not *limpness*

prefer to define *relaxation* as using only the effort appropriate to the task at hand. If you use one hundred pounds of effort to pick up a fifty-pound weight, that is tense and unrelaxed. If you use only fifty pounds of effort, then you are as relaxed as you can possibly be while still getting the job done. If you are lying in the sun with your eyes closed, listening to the birds, resting and dreaming—and expending twenty pounds of effort in your muscles—that certainly is not relaxed. It is more work than the task needs.

Many people think of limpness as the reward for exertion. They are either working all out or resting all out. But they don't monitor their internal processes as they work, to move economically, save energy, and prevent undue fatigue. The focus of the relaxation training that *Comfort at Your Computer* provides is the awareness of what makes work as efficient and easy as possible. Active relaxation is alert, soft, strong, balanced, and effective.

EXPERIMENT: POSTURAL COLLAPSE

Stand up. Notice how you are standing. Now collapse. Don't fall down on the floor. Just let your shoulders round forward and collapse. Let your head fall down. Let all your muscles sag. How does that feel? Notice that when you let your body hang on itself, certain areas experience a good deal of compression and strain. This limpness is certainly not relaxation. I would say that working relaxation—in standing up, for example—is light and free, energized and effective. As you will experience in the following chapters, real relaxation comes from strong, active, effective body use, not from limpness and collapse.

At the beginning of this chapter I defined compression as the essence of stress. When stressful situations arise, we tend to get tense and resistant. However, collapse is also a frequent response, and it too produces compression. Collapse is a process of surrender, of limp letting go. The body hangs on itself because there is no energy or will to move.

Tension and limpness are not opposites. They are two extremes of essentially the same process of inability to handle difficult situations with ease and effectiveness. As ways of life, both tension and limpness are wrong. What is needed to work at your computer comfortably and safely is a relaxed, energized, and alert way of being and moving, and that is what you are learning in this book.

• • • • • • •

The best place to practice the skill of alert relaxation is in breathing. Breathing is an odd activity. It is one of the few things we do that normally is involuntary and automatic but which is easily controlled consciously. It is a fundamental process in both rest and fight-or-flight activity. By breathing during fight-or-flight actions in a manner that is involved in rest, you can actually balance yourself between the stable state of rest and the alert state of emergency activity. You can keep your mind and body relaxed and alert and ready to deal with the stressors confronting you.

EXPERIMENT: AWARENESS OF YOUR BREATHING

I am quite sure that you are breathing as you read this. But are you aware of *how* you are breathing?

What parts of your body move as you breathe in? Do you feel movement, however great or slight, in your chest, belly, back, neck, legs, or arms? What about in your face? Or anywhere else? Where do you feel the most and least movement?

What parts of your body move as you breathe out? How do they move?

What are the movements like? Are they steady, uninterrupted and flowing? Are there stops and starts? Does one part of your breath feel more or less tense than another?

Before you learn the following breathing and relaxation exercise, you need to know some facts about how breathing actually works. The first fact is that the lungs don't do the movements of breathing. The lungs are passive sacks that allow contact between the blood and the air so that oxygen can be taken in and carbon dioxide given off.

So, if the lungs don't do the movements of breathing, what does? Imagine taking a bottle, cutting the bottom off, and taping a balloon onto the bottom. Now imagine pinching the balloon and pulling down on it. That would pull some air in through the neck of the bottle. Next imagine releasing the balloon. The balloon would spring back and the air would puff out.

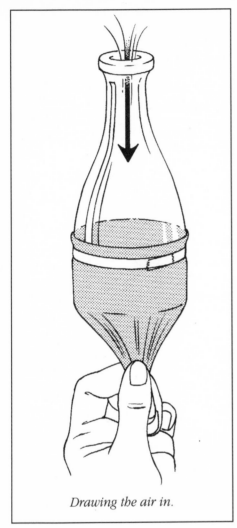

Drawing the air in.

That is how breathing works. There is a muscle called the *diaphragm*. It is a dome-shaped muscle in the chest that functions much as the balloon does with the bottle. It is dome-shaped when it is relaxed. When it tenses, it pulls tight, flattens and pushes down. That is the equivalent of the balloon being pulled down, and it is that action of the diaphragm that sucks air into the lungs.

The key point is that there is a bunch of stuff below the diaphragm—the stomach and intestines and such, and that all has to go somewhere when the diaphragm pushes down. Flesh is pretty much incompressible, so it can't be squeezed smaller. It can't move up, of course, and it also can't move down. Down below is the pelvis and the web of muscles that comprise the floor of the pelvis.

Have you ever seen a baby breathe? When babies inhale, what happens to their tummies? They expand. When the diaphragm pushes down, everything below is displaced outward, primarily to the front where the abdominal muscles can allow movement (but to some extent to the sides and back since the rib cage allows some movement there as well). This is how infants breathe, and it is the anatomically natural way to breathe, but it is not how most adults breathe.

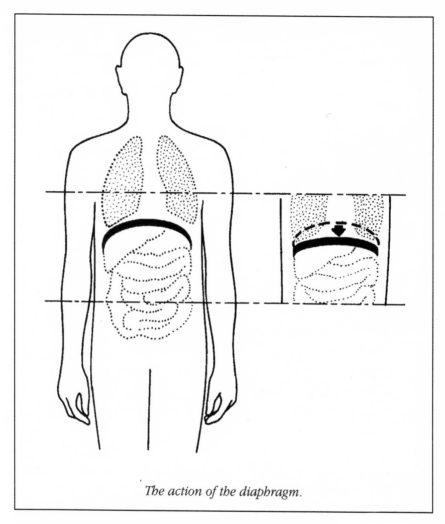

The action of the diaphragm.

Stand tall. Throw back your shoulders. Suck in your gut!

Have you ever heard this? We are taught to breathe wrong! When will someone naturally throw back their shoulders, inhale, and suck in their gut? When they are startled and scared. Americans have enshrined the fear-startle response as their ideal of beauty and strength. It is interesting to think about why this should be so, but in any case it affects everything we do.

Now you know why we started this section by paying attention to relaxing the belly. It is directly important in reducing body tension. It is also indirectly important in setting the stage for the breathing exercise that follows.

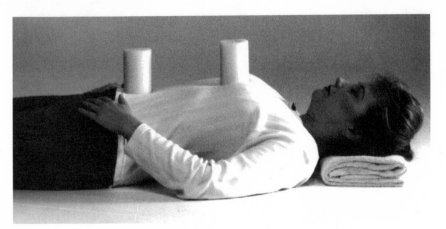

Chest breathing.

PRACTICE: BASIC BREATHING

Stand up. Now, touch your belly and notice whether you suck in your belly or let it expand when you inhale. Then touch your low back and your chest. Do they expand when you inhale?

Let your belly relax, and keep it relaxed as you inhale. Let the air fall gently down into your tummy as you inhale, and let your tummy expand. Your belly should be the focal point of your breathing, but it is important to let your chest and low back also swell gently as you inhale.

Compressing your belly as you inhale rigidifies your chest, belly, and back and creates a lot of tension in your body. However, if you have gotten used to sucking in your gut as you inhale, breathing in a more relaxed manner will feel strange. At first you may even have the strange sensation that it feels physically better to breathe from your belly, but it is so unfamiliar that it feels uncomfortable to breathe more comfortably.

If expanding and inhaling is difficult, at first you may have to deliberately push your belly out as you inhale just to get the rhythm. Later you can give up this extra effort.

Some people find it very hard to figure out how to either expand or push out their bellies. A way to help with this is to lie down on your back, with pillows under your head and knees, put a fist sized

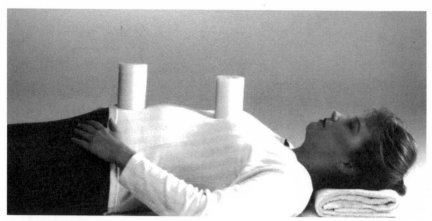

Belly breathing.

stone (or something similar) on your belly just below your belly button, and concentrate on raising the stone by inhaling.

Once you have found out how to expand and inhale, try standing and breathing in through your nose and out through your mouth. Let your whole torso relax and open, so that the air comes in and falls gently down to your pelvis. (Of course the *air* stays in your lungs, but this image will help you feel the *movement* all the way down through your body.)

Breathing in through your nose and out through your mouth is useful for two reasons. It changes the absolutely ordinary process of breathing into something new, which helps you stay focused on it. Also, it is a bridge between an inner and an outer focus. Normally you breathe out through your mouth only when you are talking or expending physical effort. Both those tasks are directed outward into the world. The breathing exercise focuses on what you are doing inside your body, but its purpose is to cultivate an inward relaxation that will allow effective functioning out in the world.

Ideally you should relax your belly and breathe from there all the time. However, breathing in through your nose and out through your mouth is just for this exercise. In daily life, you should breathe normally, in and out through your nose.

Breathing and expanding is very relaxing. Breathing is supposed to be a gentle, internal massage, and it is very comfortable when it is. Most people, when they try walking or doing other movements in the overall state of pelvic release and soft breathing, feel that their movement is easier, better balanced, more graceful, more coordinated, and much more solidly connected to the ground. You will find that this new physical state allows you to work at the computer in a physically freer and more relaxed way.

In addition to the physical benefits, this internal physical softness also creates a psychological state of relaxed alertness. Negative feelings such fear, anger, anxiety, confusion, and so on always involve some form of twisting and constriction or collapse in muscles, breathing, posture, and movement. Breathing in an open way is the opposite of this constriction and serves to counteract emotional stress. As an aside, I should say that negative feelings are a natural part of our human makeup and are often important to explore. However, since negative feelings are one factor in repetitive strain injuries, you need to find a way to settle these feelings while you are working at your computer.

EXPERIMENT: SLUGS IN YOUR FACE

You will need a partner for this experiment in using breathing as a means of reducing emotional stress. You and your partner should stand facing each other. First you need some stress to overcome, and a simple image and movement can help you find some. Your partner was out in their garden last night, picking slugs off lettuce plants, and they saved all the slugs. Now, have your partner rub a handful of the slugs all over your face.

What do you do when your partner rubs the (imaginary) slugs in your face? What happens to your breathing? Does your posture change? Do you stay relaxed and alert? Do you tense up and pull away? Or something else? What do you do in your face? The imaginary slugs coupled with the real physical intrusion of the rubbing almost always make people very squeamish and uncomfortable. Most people pull away, grimace, tense up, and restrict their breathing in a variety of ways.

Now, consciously and deliberately relax your belly and breathing as your partner rubs the slugs into your face. Breathe in through your nose and out through your mouth, keeping your breathing soft and steady. How does that affect the way you respond? Most people experience that it vastly reduces the emotional discomfort of the exercise. Many people even find that an intrusion that was very uncomfortable at first becomes quite trivial when they maintain their focus and relaxation. This state of alert relaxation is what I call *being centered*.

A little caution might be important in this experiment. Many people have been abused or assaulted in various ways, and they may have extreme reactions to being touched or intruded upon. If you don't want to be touched, simply don't do the experiment. Honor your own feelings and needs. Or if you want to structure the experiment to be less threatening, you might have your partner stand back five or ten feet and just throw tissues at you. This is usually much less stressful but still stressful enough to be valuable as a practice.

Of course, at the other extreme, some people are used to violent contact sports and so on, and they don't find having slugs rubbed in their faces at all stressful. If you are in that category, you might consider consulting with your partner and figuring out something that would be stressful enough to be productive as an exercise for you. Remember that the exercise has to be safe and that your partner has to be comfortable enough with their role in the exercise to do it.

• • • • • • •

Emotions are physical events in the body. Do you think you could be emotionally angry and at the same time physically soft, gentle, and relaxed? Could you be emotionally depressed and physically energetic, alert, and comfortable? Emotions are physical events, and *feelings* are what those physical events feel like to the person undergoing them. The point is that if emotions are physical events, you can control emotions physically. You can replace the physical events of anxiety with the physical events of alert relaxation.

If you use the physical techniques for pelvic softening and breathing when you feel anxious about some performance situation, you will find that you are able to create and maintain a relaxed and alert mental and physical state. You will find that whatever difficulty you face will feel much less threatening and uncomfortable, and this will enable you to deal with the situation more effectively, thereby further reducing the anxiety you feel.

• • • • • • •

Along with breathing comes speaking, and there is an emotional component to the act of speaking. In the first edition of this book, I didn't include any exercises for speaking in a relaxed and safe manner. But then came dictation software, and people started using dictation to reduce the amount of keyboarding they needed to do. However, many people who use dictation software in an effort to reduce strain on their wrists experience vocal strain. They simply trade one strain for another. The problem is that people who are fundamentally stressed will create strain in whatever part of the body they happen to be using.

EXPERIMENT: ICK AND AHH

Stand up, feel your breathing. Count out loud from one to ten, and notice what parts of your body are involved in breathing and vocalizing. More than noticing just what parts move, notice how they feel as they move. Are your lips and tongue tense? Do you speak in a sharp or clipped manner?

Now, try saying "Rat guts, ick!" And for contrast say "Ice cream, ahh!"

Say "ick" and "ahh." Feel how your throat and mouth tense when you say "ick" and how they get softer and smoother when you say "ahh."

The expressions "ick" and "ahh" are very interesting. They simultaneously create and reflect the body processes of repulsion and enjoyment. "Ick" has sharp edges and creates constriction. "Ahh" has round edges and creates softness.

How do you talk when you talk to your co-workers or use your dictation software? Is it more like ick or more like ahh? Is your throat tense? Are you tense, perhaps from irritation with your computer or from stress at approaching deadlines? If you tense your throat and your voice, hour after hour of speaking that way will produce strain and damage.

PRACTICE: RELAXED SPEAKING

Try counting aloud again. Let the feeling of ahh come into your speech. Let your tongue and lips be soft, pliable, and gentle. Let your throat be loose and open. Of course, you should let your breathing be gentle and full. And make sure to talk in a slow and languid way.

Later on you can practice talking more rapidly but maintaining the same feeling of softness.

How would it feel to say urgent things in a gentle and soft way? You might find that would considerably reduce the anxiety you feel.

Taking care to breathe and talk gently will do a lot to relax your whole body, and it will also prevent vocal strain from using dictation software. Actually, every body part and every movement influences every other part or movement. As you continue with exercises on postural stability and ease, you will find they will help you reduce vocal strain as well.

Softening the belly, breathing, and voice is the beginning of an overall balancing of the whole body. We've started with the core of the body, and the next step in our journey will be to move outward along the spinal column.

KEY POINTS

- Releasing tension is the *undoing* part of overcoming stress. Finding a state of energized support is the *doing* part. The two elements of releasing and supporting are the basis for safe, comfortable computer use.
- A key to reducing stress is softening the core of your body and your breathing. Feel your breathing. Let your belly gently expand as you inhale. Let your chest and back open as well.
- It is OK to let your belly relax. You don't have to believe the social messages that tension and constriction look good. Remember that constricting the core of your body results in weakness, imbalance, and discomfort.
- *Emotions* are physical events in the body. *Feelings* are what the events feel like to the person undergoing them. Since emotions are physical events, you can control emotions physically. You can replace the physical events of stress with the physical events of alert relaxation.

- Keeping your breathing soft and free will help you stay relaxed in stressful situations. Tightening your breathing will make the situations difficult to handle.
- Keeping your voice relaxed and free will help you prevent vocal strain.

BALANCING YOUR
PELVIS AND SPINAL COLUMN

Tensing your muscles unnecessarily is just one way of overworking them. Sitting in a position that requires the wrong muscles to work at holding up your body is another way of overworking your muscles. In addition to simple relaxation, efficient postural support is also necessary to relieve computer stress.

An understanding of the body's architecture is crucial. Bones are like the support beams in a building. When the weight of your body falls squarely through your bones to the surface supporting your body, then your muscles don't have to work very much. In addition, your body will be in a position of balance that allows free, uncompressed movement in your breathing and your joints. However, when your body leans off the vertical line, your muscles must work overtime to hold your body up, and your joints will be loaded in imbalanced ways. There will be considerable structural strain and fatigue. Postural balancing is a process of eliminating the waste of energy involved in misusing the body's system of support beams.

As an example, think about a tall flagpole being held up by guy lines on all sides. As long as the pole stays vertical, only slight adjustments and minor force will be necessary to keep it up. Most of the pole's weight will be transferred vertically through its own length into the ground. But if it starts to tip off vertical, a lot of force will be needed to keep it from continuing its movement and falling. In the same way, a vertical postural support pattern allows the bones to support the weight of the body with as little effort as possible. Sitting in a vertically balanced posture vastly decreases the muscular effort involved in maintaining the sitting position.

In one way, the flagpole is a good image of postural balance, but in another way it is a very poor image. A flagpole is an inert object, but people are not inert objects. Many people make the mistake of thinking that good posture is really stiff and motionless. "Posture" sounds a lot like "post," and very often people believe that good posture is like being a sturdy, upright, immovable post. They think you get into the right position and you stay there, but that is a prescription for static holding and postural strain.

In fact, good posture is a fluid, dynamic *process*. Good posture is a continuing action, or more precisely, a continuing series of actions—of

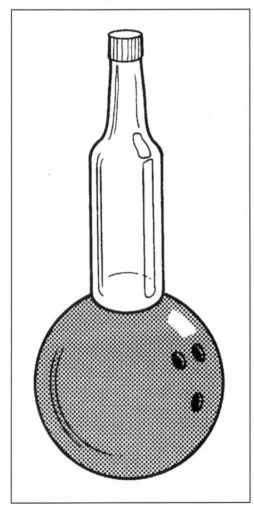

small movements of adjustment around a central line of balance. Only dead people have "good posture" in the static, unmoving sense. When you sit "still" at your computer, you are actually in constant movement. Sitting is really a process of movement.

The flagpole image also suggests an unfortunate idea of the nature of postural adjustment. A leaning flagpole is brought back to a vertical position by lengthening the guy wires on the side the pole leans toward and shortening the guy wires on the side it leans away from. Many people think of postural adjustment as a merely mechanical process like straightening up a leaning flagpole. They think that doing strengthening exercises to shorten slack muscles and doing flexibility exercises to stretch tight muscles will bring the body to a vertical alignment. However, posture is a dynamic process of movement, and movements are *actions*. Whether we are doing the movements with conscious awareness or not, on some mind/body level movements are choices. Movements are part of the style and meaning of our lives, and therefore postural change has to involve awareness and choice. We have to *understand* and *feel* how we are moving and why we move that way in order to change our movements most effectively.

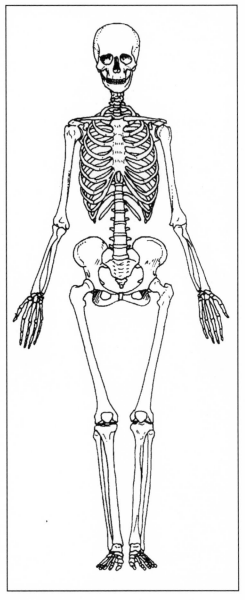

Let's start by examining the movement processes of the core of the body. Consider how you balance your spinal column on your pelvis. It is very much like balancing a bottle upright on a bowling ball. The spinal column is like a bottle, and the pelvis is like a bowling ball. If the bottle is placed just exactly right on the bowling ball, it will balance and stay upright. However, once it is balanced, if the bowling ball rolls underneath it, the bottle will fall off the ball. The spinal column, of course cannot fall off the pelvis. However, if the pelvis rotates forward, the lower back will be dragged forward into a swaybacked position; and if the pelvis rotates backward, the lower back will be dragged backward into a slumped position.

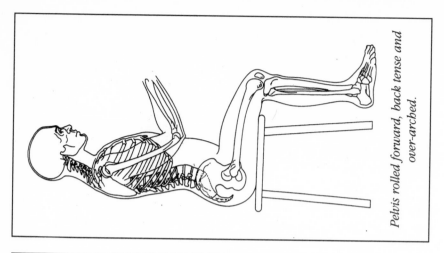

Pelvis rolled forward, back tense and over-arched.

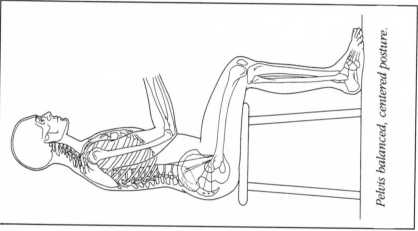

Pelvis balanced, centered posture.

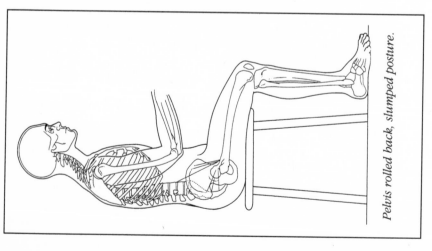

Pelvis rolled back, slumped posture.

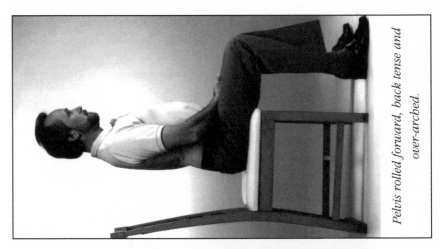

Pelvis rolled forward, back tense and over-arched.

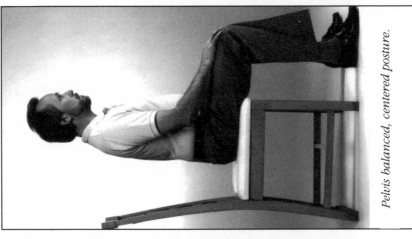

Pelvis balanced, centered posture.

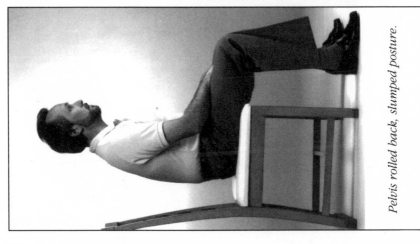

Pelvis rolled back, slumped posture.

EXPERIMENT: PELVIC ROTATION

There is a simple experiment that will help you feel how your pelvis and spinal column operate together to provide postural support. Find a firm chair with a flat, level seat pan (the part of the chair you sit on). Some chairs have bucket-shaped or very soft seat pans or seat pans that slant back, and these chairs force you to adopt a posture that conforms to their design. However, in order to do this experiment, you will need to be sitting in a chair that offers neutral support. If your chair is too soft and cushy or forces you to lean way back, it won't work for this experiment. If you don't have a chair with a flat, level seat pan, you can use an ordinary chair with a minimal tilt or bucket—such as a library chair or a cafeteria chair. Simply fill in the rear edge of the seat pan with folded towels to create a flat and level surface to sit on.

Sit without leaning against the back support, and try slumping down and sitting up straight. By slumping, I mean a movement in which you let your body collapse downward. Your shoulders go down but not very much forward. Some people, when they are asked to slump, will bend forward from the waist and drop their head down toward their knees. That is not what I mean by slumping.

Notice that when you slump, your pelvis rotates backward. The stack of vertebrae has no foundation on which to rest, and it curves and slumps down. (The pelvis can be thought of as a bowl that contains the guts, and "backward" is the direction in which the bowl would rotate to spill out the guts behind the body.) Notice that when you roll your pelvis forward, your body moves up out of the slump to an erect sitting posture. And if you continue rolling your pelvis forward past the point of erect posture, your back arches into a swayback position.

Contrary to what most people believe, straightening up from a slump is accomplished by rolling the pelvis forward not by throwing the shoulders back or by straightening the back. Movements of the shoulders or back are extra movements that use muscles unnecessarily and waste energy. If you aren't sure about this, slump and feel how your pelvis rolls back. Now, without moving your pelvis at all, try to sit up by moving your shoulders. It can't be done.

Some people find it difficult to do the movement of pelvic rotation while sitting, but practicing it in another position can be easier. Get down onto all fours, standing on your hands and knees, with your arms and legs pretty much vertical (but not locked) and straight underneath you. Now, gently arch your back, letting it sag down into a swayback position— like a horse that has had too many heavy riders. And then hump your back up—like an angry cat. Move slowly and gently back and forth

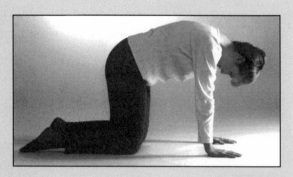

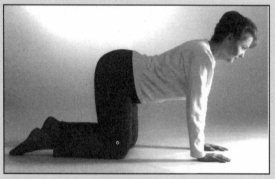

Rolling the pelvis forward and back.

from the arched to the humped position, feeling how your pelvis rolls and your spinal column follows the rolling. Once you have felt the movement clearly, try it again in the sitting position.

EXPERIMENT: FINDING THE HIP SOCKET

The rotation movement of your pelvis centers around your hip sockets. The hip is not the bony edge that you feel on your side just below your belt. That is the lip of the pelvic bowl. The hip is a joint, the leg's equivalent of the shoulder, and the hip socket itself is deep in the upper part of the leg. Stand up on one leg, and raise the other in front of you. Where the fold is in your leg, that is where your hip is.

Rolling the pelvis forward and back.

There are two very different sets of muscles that will rotate your pelvis forward. Using one produces strain and imbalance in your body, and using the other produces balance, power, and ease. To understand this, consider that there are basically two ways to tip a bowl forward—lifting the rear edge or lowering the front edge. Which edge of the bowl moves determines where the axis of rotation is, and which edge of the pelvis is the focus of movement determines whether pelvic rotation will be an easy movement or a strain.

Most people sit up "straight" by arching their backs. This is done by using the muscles along the surface of the back to pull up on the rear edge of the pelvis. However, it creates tension and discomfort, and this is why everyone will sit up "straight" for a minute when exhorted to and then give it up as uncomfortable. The most effective and comfortable way of rotating your pelvis forward involves using muscles deep in the core of the body rather than muscles along the surface of the back. Those muscles are the psoas (pronounced *so-as*) and the iliacus. These deep, internal muscles cause a movement that drops the front edge of the pelvis and creates a very strong and comfortable physical organization of the pelvis and spinal column.

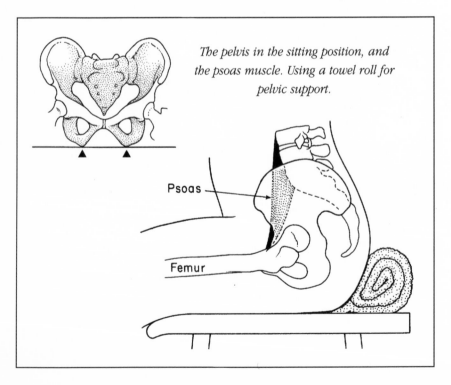

The pelvis in the sitting position, and the psoas muscle. Using a towel roll for pelvic support.

Psoas

Femur

EXPERIMENT: FINDING PROPER PELVIC ROTATION

How can you find this new way of moving your pelvis? Sit toward the front edge of your firm flat chair, with your back not touching the backrest. Keep your knees spread comfortably apart, your feet flat on the ground and your lower legs perpendicular to the ground (not tucked underneath you or stretched way out in front). Just for contrast, start by moving the wrong way, lifting from the back of your pelvis. Roll your pelvis forward by arching your back and lifting your back pockets up toward your shoulders. Notice that the movement takes place in your back around your waist. Notice also how tense this makes your lower back. Most people will tend to pull their shoulder blades down as well as their back pockets up, and this will spread the tension up through the whole back.

Now, let's find the better way. Slump down. The new movement will be very low in your body, coming from deep in the pelvis, around your hip sockets. Notice that when you sit slumped your genitals point upwards. Roll your pelvis forward by moving your genitals forward and down so that they point toward the floor. You will almost have the feeling that you are going to sit on top of your genitals.

It is important to keep your knees and feet apart a bit as you try to find the proper way of rotating your pelvis. If you press your legs together, that will create tension in the pelvis/back unit and prevent free movement of your pelvis and spinal column.

Notice in the illustrations of the balanced sitting posture that when the pelvis is balanced the body leans just a bit forward. Roll your pelvis to sit up and then lean a bit backward. What does that do? Most people will feel that moving off the line of balance creates tension in their backs and breathing. When you were a kid, did you try to balance your spoon on the lip of your cereal bowl at breakfast? Balancing on your pelvis is just like that. If you find just the right weight placement, the balance will be easy, and if you move off that placement, you won't be balanced.

You will know you are doing the movement right when you move easily into an erect sitting posture. Your back and shoulders will not be actively engaged in muscular work but will move in a soft and relaxed way, simply as a result of the pelvic rotation.

I should address an issue here that may be important to some people. In Chapter 4, as part of softening your breathing, I had you release the tension in your genital and anal sphincter muscles. Here I have defined a new sitting position by the orientation of the genitals. Many people have been sexually abused or in other ways made to feel very uncomfortable about noticing, feeling, or mentioning the pelvic area of the body. However, it is just another part of the body, like your elbow. And the proper use of the pelvis and pelvic floor muscles is crucial in developing the body architecture required for comfortable sitting. If you find talking about this difficult, please take an honest look at the source of your discomfort, and don't give up on learning to be comfortable, strong, and safe in your body.

This new way of sitting places the bones of the pelvis and spinal column in the architecturally optimal alignment. The weight of the body is on a vertical line through the head and torso. It goes squarely through the sitbones into the chair. (Your sitbones are the ischial tuberosities, the two pointy bones in your bottom that press into whatever you sit on. If you aren't sure where your sitbones are, sit for a while on a flat concrete surface, and you will certainly begin to notice the hard bones pressing into the hard concrete.)

I try not to use the word *straight* in talking about sitting. I prefer the word *vertical*. Sitting *straight* has connotations of being tense, held in, in a military posture. Sitting vertically is a comfortable and relaxed way of being in your body. Sitting vertically has an upward-opening and lengthening feeling to it, like a flower growing toward the sun, with its roots joining the earth. Your body gently lengthens upward rather than sagging or slumping, and the upward vertical lengthening allows your body's weight to fall squarely onto the support surface below your body. I call this *centered* sitting.

Vertical does not mean straight like a ruler. In a simple sitting or standing position, the body is vertical when all the body's normal curves average out so that the skeleton directs the body's weight directly into the ground. There is a bit of forward lean in proper vertical sitting (as shown in the drawing of the balanced pelvis). Sitting with just a bit of forward lean moves the body's weight along the thigh, away from the rear edge of the body. Bringing the center of gravity forward delivers the body's weight into the ground in a more stable and balanced way.

Many people believe that good sitting should be straight and military, with a ninety degree angle of the thighs and torso. Many other people believe that good sitting should involve leaning back so the body's weight falls onto the chair's backrest. Both of these postures are problematic. However, in order to understand why, you will have to have more experience with the way the body balances itself, so we will put off discussing these ideas about posture until Chapter 11.

Sitting upright by using your psoas and iliacus to balance your body can vastly decrease the feeling of strain and fatigue caused by computer work. It makes long periods of sitting at your computer more comfortable and allows you to utilize more of your energy for productive work instead of wasting it in physical discomfort.

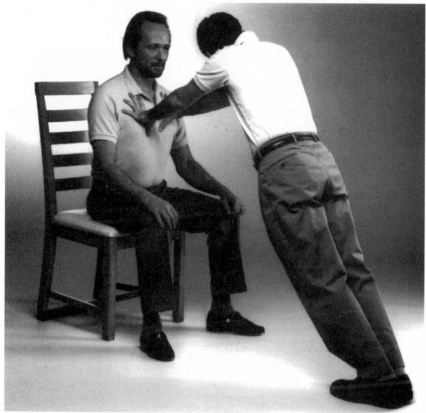

With a centered sitting posture, the model is able to take the pusher's whole body weight and stay relaxed. Most people should start off with less pressure.

EXPERIMENT: CHEST PUSH SITTING TEST

There is a test that will help you determine whether you are sitting well. You will need a partner to help with this. Your partner's job will be to push on your chest, and your job will be to maintain your sitting posture and not be pushed over backward. Sit toward the front of your flat, neutral chair. Don't lean back against the backrest. Have your partner sit on another chair in front of you.

First, sit up *straight*, like a model of social correctness. Suck in your guts and throw back your shoulders. Have your partner push on your chest, with a steady pressure, and not with extreme force. In this sitting posture, can you resist the pressure?

Now, slump down, and then come up to a good sitting posture by rolling your pelvis forward in the proper way. Relax your belly and breathe. Have your partner push again. If you are sitting correctly, you will feel the pressure of the push somehow get deflected from a line going straight back through your chest into a line moving diagonally down and back. The pressure will actually press you into the chair and stabilize your posture, and you will feel that you are not working very hard to achieve the stability. Of course, there are limits to how much pressure you can absorb. Your partner should be reasonable and not push too hard.

Now that you have felt how to align the pelvis and spinal column through using the psoas and iliacus, you are ready to learn how to maintain that alignment without even using them very much. Think about putting a brick under a car wheel to keep the car from rolling. That is just what we are going to do to keep the pelvis/spinal column stabilized.

PRACTICE: TOWEL SITTING

You need a bath towel for this. If it is really large and thick, it won't work. And likewise, if it is thin and skimpy, it won't work. Take an ordinary bath towel and fold it in half widthwise. Then fold it in half lengthwise. Then roll it up, not too tight and hard, but also not too loose.

Sitting in your comfortable, well-aligned position, lean forward and get your weight off your bottom and onto your feet. Raise your sitbones off the chair a few inches, put the towel roll underneath your tailbone, and then sit back down onto the towel roll. It is important that the towel be positioned under your tail-bone not under your sitbones. Your sitbones must still rest on the chair surface.

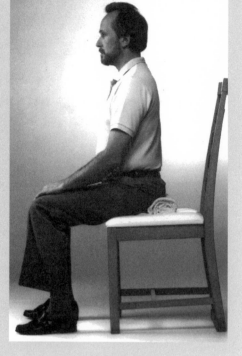

Then come back to your vertical sitting posture. If you have the towel positioned right, you will feel your tail-bone resting on it and the towel supporting your whole spinal column and torso. Most people feel lighter and freer when they sit with a towel roll for support. They feel that the effort they usually expend on holding their bod-ies up simply isn't needed.

Towel sitting.

You can understand why this towel roll is so comfortable if you think of the pelvis as a two legged stool. There is a reason why stools have three legs (or four). It is very simple. Two legged stools fall over. Well, the pelvis is essentially a two legged stool. When you sit down, the two sitbones are all that contact the surface of the chair, and that is an essentially unstable arrangement. It takes muscular effort to hold the pelvis in position, and people usually use the back muscles to hold the pelvis in position. Those are the wrong muscles, and they tire quickly. In trying to reduce the effort, people slump until their bodies hang stably on their ligaments. A better way to cre-ate stability is to use the psoas and iliacus muscles to hold the pelvis in position. Better still is using the muscles to position the pelvis properly and then filling in the gap between the tailbone and the chair surface. This in effect provides a third leg for the stool and reduces even the work the psoas and iliacus need to do.

You need to be able to find the stable, vertical posture through your own body actions, but once you know how to create a balanced sitting posture on your own, you can use a towel roll to support yourself in this posture. It may be a startling idea, but you can work at a computer most comfortably if you sit up without leaning against a backrest at all. Proper body alignment coupled with proper pelvic support is the key to proper sitting at the computer. (I do recommend having and occasionally using a backrest, as will be discussed later.) There is, however, more to correct sitting than just proper pelvic alignment, and as we continue with the tour of the body, you will gain a clearer understanding of how to sit most comfortably.

Sitting properly is very comfortable, but I want to emphasize that you shouldn't sit even this way for too long. You should *keep moving*. Keep moving! I can't say that enough. The body is not designed to maintain static postures. Even the best sitting posture will become uncomfortable if you don't keep moving. In Chapters 12 and 14, we will work with movement breaks you can use while at work.

I should also mention that the sitting posture you are learning is designed for alert functioning at an upright task. It isn't necessarily the one-and-only correct way to sit. You probably wouldn't want to watch TV in the same position in which you type. Watching TV doesn't demand the mental alertness or physical effort required by computer use. How you should sit depends on what you are doing.

EXPERIMENT: STRESS AND SITTING

Remember the Slugs in Your Face experiment in the section on breathing (Chapter 4)? Try the same test, sitting down this time. Add to the relaxation of your belly and breathing the strong, balanced centered way of sitting. Most people experience that this relaxed as well as alert and strong way of sitting is even more effective in reducing the emotional discomfort of the exercise. Many people find that beyond feeling just relaxed, they now feel alert and energized and ready to face the intrusion.

The way you organize your body is also the way your organize your mind. The physical/psychological feeling of stability and strength produced by proper sitting and breathing is very helpful in handling the emotional stresses that inevitably are part of work.

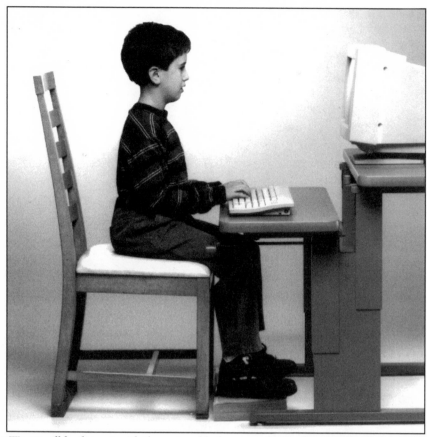

We are all built to sit with the natural balance and ease shown here by my son. If we have lost it, we can relearn it.

Take another look at the picture of my son, in Chapter 4. Notice that he is naturally sitting in just the way we have been practicing. I did not have to teach him that. He sat that way naturally, and most children do. It is our birthright as the graceful animals we are. Most of us have lost it, but we can relearn it.

Sitting right is the core of safety and comfort in computer use. You don't have to sit scrunched and uncomfortable. By paying attention to how you sit, you can preserve your health and work comfortably at your computer.

KEY POINTS

- Efficient postural support is important. When the weight of your body falls squarely through your bones to the surface supporting your body, then your muscles will not have to work very much. Your body will be in a position of balance, which will allow free, uncompressed breathing and movement.

- Good posture is not static. It is a fluid, dynamic process of continuing small movements of adjustment around a central line of balance.

- Postural movements are part of the style and meaning of our lives, and therefore postural change has to involve awareness and choice.

- The pelvis is the foundation for the spinal column. Finding and maintaining proper pelvis/spinal column balance is the core of good posture. In order to achieve effortless and efficient sitting, roll your pelvis forward by using the psoas and iliacus muscles.

- Place a towel roll under your tailbone to support your pelvis and reduce the effort it takes to maintain good sitting posture.

- With proper body alignment and pelvic support, it will be most comfortable to sit at the computer without leaning against a backrest.

- Maintaining a physically strong, balanced posture will help you stay mentally relaxed and focused in stressful situations.

GETTING TO THE HEART OF IT

So far we have looked at the belly, pelvis, and spinal column. The way you use your chest is also very important, both in relaxation and in body positioning.

EXPERIMENT: CHEST ELEVATION

What is the relationship between your belly and your chest? Stand up, and try elevating (raising or puffing up) your chest.

What happens in your back when you elevate your chest? What do you do with your low back and the area around your shoulder blades? Notice that you elevate your chest by tensing and arching your back. Some people arch their backs directly, and some arch their backs by pulling their shoulders back and drawing their shoulder blades together. In any case, your ribs are attached to your spinal column, and you move your ribs by moving your spine. You can think of your ribs as similar to the ribs of a paper fan. When your spine arches, your ribs fan out.

Can you relax your belly at the same time as you elevate your chest? It is possible, but it is an odd thing to do. Most people automatically tense their bellies when they tense their backs to elevate their chests.

How does elevating your chest affect your breathing? Can you breathe softly, easily and fully when you puff up your chest? Notice that tensing your chest tenses and restricts your breathing, just the opposite of what you want for comfortable computer use.

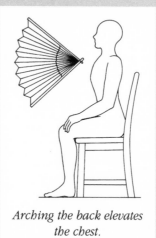

Arching the back elevates the chest.

Many people try to avoid slumping at the computer by "sitting tall." They do this by elongating and elevating the front of their bodies and tensing the back of their bodies, but that prevents soft breathing. They think they are improving their posture, but what they are really doing is compressing their bodies. When your pelvis and spinal column are balanced, and your belly and breathing are relaxed, then your chest will soften and fall from the elevated position into its natural alignment.

At first, many people feel that they are caving in their chests when they sit in this softly natural way. People often feel like "gorillas" or "Neanderthals," but after a while they get used to it. As a general rule, we equate "habitual" with "correct." Whatever we normally do *feels* like the right thing to do—even when it isn't. In order to learn a new and better way of doing something, we often have to do what we intellectually know is right, even when it feels wrong, and keep practicing it until it starts feeling right.

• • • • • • • •

Aside from the positioning of the chest, another very important aspect of body use has to do with a particular *feeling* in the chest. This can be experienced through working with imagery and body responses.

PRACTICE: SMILING HEART

Everyone has something or someone—perhaps a friend, a lover, a child, a flower, a work of art—something that when they think of it makes their heart smile.

Stand with your eyes closed, and spend a few moments thinking about whatever it is that makes your heart smile. What happens in your body? How is your chest affected? What happens to your breathing? What sensations do you feel flowing through you?

Most people experience a softening and warmth in their chests, and a freeing up throughout their bodies.

These sensations of being "warm-hearted" or "tender-hearted" are the bodily manifestations of love or compassion. If you stop to think about it, you will notice that very often we use physical language to describe emotional qualities. We talk about someone being *stiff-necked* or *warm-hearted* or having *guts*. There is a wisdom to this. Our emotional feelings are rooted in our physical life.

Most people have accepted that the mind can produce illness in the body. Very few people have thought about the fact the body controls the mind just as much as the mind controls the body. In fact, they are one and the same. Mind and body are just two sides of the same coin. Working with your muscle tone, breathing and posture is a direct way of making emotional and behavioral changes.

EXPERIMENT: HATRED

Try imagining someone who is a constant source of irritation and obstruction, perhaps a boss who constantly belittles you, or a co-worker who always shirks his own work but tries to take credit for work you have done. You have tried everything you can think of to resolve the situation, but the jerk just makes fun of you for trying. Let yourself feel irritation and resentment. Even hatred.

What happens in your body? What do you do in your breathing? In your chest and your posture as a whole?

Negative feelings such as fear and anger produce constriction, hardness and imbalance in breathing and the chest, and this will result in stressful, antagonistic ways of acting.

Feelings take place in the body. By observing and changing our bodies, we can understand and change what we feel.

EXPERIMENT: BACK TO THE SLUGS

Let's try the slugs-in-the-face exercise again. Remember the earlier versions in Chapters 4 and 5? Sit in front of your partner. Relax your breathing and align your pelvis as you did then. And this time also stay with the image that makes your heart smile.

What happens to your feelings of being intruded on or threatened? How do you feel about your "enemy" when you keep yourself relaxed, strong, and compassionate?

Many people report that when they do these three body processes all together, not only do they not feel threatened by their slug-masher, but they feel very warm toward her or him. Moreover, they find that this state of being allows them to dominate the interaction instead of feeling intruded on and pushed around.

Creating the sensation of softness and love in the chest is a way of replacing antagonistic feelings with more harmonious feelings. In this physical state, you will indeed feel loving and act in genuinely loving ways.

Some people are uncomfortable with the idea of softening their chests rather than hardening and elevating them. Our culture's image of strength and beauty includes an elevated and hardened chest. Think of a "manly man," with tight muscles and an expanded chest. Think of a beautiful ballerina, with a long line and an elevated chest. Remember the drawings from the advertisements (in Chapter 4). However, as you experienced in the exercise on chest elevation, people pay the price of tension and discomfort for this hardening and elevating. And rather than producing strength, it actually causes weakness and instability.

EXPERIMENT: CHEST PUSH AND PUFFED UP CHEST

Try the chest push exercise described in Chapter 5 again. Start by stabilizing and aligning your body as well as you can, and then harden and elevate your chest. Get tough and strong!

Now have your partner push on your chest as she or he did before. What happens? You will undoubtedly be pushed right over. Notice that elevating your chest makes you top heavy and unstable. The very thing that society believes is a sign of strength is a cause of weakness.

This weakness is emotional as well as physical. Try the slugs-in-the-face exercise again. But this time, instead of relaxing, puff up your chest. Grit your teeth. Get strong and determined. You will resist the insult and intrusion of having slugs rubbed into your face!

What happens? What do you do? What do you feel? Most people find that the intrusion feels much worse when they tense up to resist it. They find themselves shying away, or getting angry. They find themselves disliking their partner.

The idea that love or compassion is a source of strength is not philosophy. It is simply a statement of the fact that your body works best in states of relaxation and freedom. Fear, anger, and other negative emotions produce tension and imbalance in your body.

At first sight, the idea of warm-heartedness might seem pretty far removed from the topic of using your body correctly when you work at a computer. However, along with pelvic softening and positioning, this physical state of love is helpful in overcoming feelings of pressure and anxiety that arise as you attempt to handle complex work activities under deadlines and other pressures.

Beyond simple work pressures, interpersonal pressures also are very stressful. Knowing how to create a loving state and act from it can be very helpful in smoothing out the interpersonal conflicts that often arise in work situations. If you can respond with an open heart to your antagonist, you have a chance of establishing a more positive connection between both of you. This skill offers an important means of changing the atmosphere of the workplace. If you can become calmer and more accepting, that will exert some leverage on the behavior of everyone around you. Think how different work would be if everyone in the office chose to use these body awareness tools to create a more harmonious workplace.

KEY POINTS

- Your ribcage is attached to and supported by your spinal column. You elevate your chest by tensing and arching your back, which tenses and restricts your belly and your breathing. Let your chest stay soft and find its natural position of relaxed balance.
- The sensations in the chest of being "warm hearted" are the bodily manifestations of compassion, and they soften and free up the chest. Negative feelings such as fear and anger produce constriction, hardness and imbalance in breathing and the chest. In order to create a free and balanced posture, it is important to maintain harmonious feelings.
- Mind and body are one and the same. Working with your muscle tone, breathing, and posture is a direct way of making emotional and behavioral changes.
- Creating the sensation of softness and love in your chest during stressful situations is a way of feeling more harmonious and acting in more loving ways.

7

GAINING EASE IN YOUR
HANDS, ARMS AND SHOULDERS

Strain in the wrist and arm is a significant, specific problem for many computer users. Typing on a keyboard involves both static holding and dynamic activity. Holding your arms in position over the keyboard is static work, and the continuous movement of your fingers is dynamic work. However, arm strain is not simple. It can be caused by mistakes in your overall body posture or by specific mistakes in your ways of using your arms.

WHOLE BODY

The first thing to know about your arm is that it is designed for mobility. If the shoulder joint were a full ball-and-socket joint, with the ball of the humerus (the upper arm bone) fitting into a deep semi-spherical hollow of bone, that would narrow the angle of its possible movements. Instead, the head of the humerus rests on a shallow dish. Rather than being held in place by a deep socket, the humerus is held in position by muscles and ligaments. Because of this arrangement, the arm can move and swing freely in many different directions.

The dish that the humerus fits into is part of the shoulder blade. The shoulder blade is essentially a curved bony plate simply placed against the rear surface of the rib cage and held there by muscles. The shoulder blade itself can move

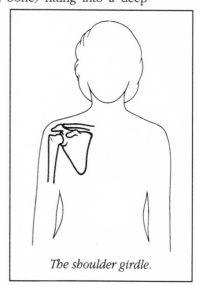

The shoulder girdle.

around quite freely. The shoulder blade attaches to the collar bone by a joint at the top of the shoulder, and the collar bone is also quite movable. The shoulder blade and the collar bone form the attachment for the arm, and the whole arrangement is called the *shoulder girdle*.

Your shoulder blade sits against the back of your rib cage, and your collar bone attaches to the front of your ribcage (at your breastbone). This is the important point: your ribs attach to and are moved by your spinal column, and your collar bone and shoulder blade are also positioned largely by your spinal column. Your spinal column in turn is positioned by your pelvis. If your pelvis-spinal column unit is not balanced, then your arms will be held in an imbalanced position, and this will produce inefficiency and strain in every movement your arms make. Therefore, pelvic balance is the beginning of arm comfort. Once your pelvis and spinal column are balanced well, the most efficient and comfortable position for your arms will become clear.

EXPERIMENT: PELVIC ROTATION AND ARM USE

Sit on a flat chair without touching the backrest. Now slump. Feel how your pelvis rolls back and your torso collapses. Notice how your collar bones and shoulders roll forward and down. From this position, try raising your arms forward and up in front of you to about shoulder height. Notice how your arms feel. Is the movement smooth and steady, or is it jerky? Do your arms feel light and free or heavy and constrained? Most people feel that the range of motion of their arms is restricted. They feel that the tops of their upper arms hit a "barrier" and that there is considerable tension in their necks.

Next adopt a straight "military" posture, throwing back your shoulders, sucking in your gut, and "straightening" your back. Try raising your arms again. What happens to the quality and feel of the movement? Most people, when they raise their arms from this position, feel that the underside of their arms near their armpits is pulled down. Again the arms cannot move freely upward, and people generally experience considerable tension in the middle of the back and neck as well.

Sit in the vertical, balanced, centered way you practiced in Chapter 5. Try pulling your shoulders up and then back. Notice what that extra effort feels like. Then let your shoulders settle into their position of natural support and ease. Let your shoulders relax.

Let them settle into the position in which they are naturally and easily supported by the pelvis/spinal column unit. They will not be held up around your ears, nor will they be pulled back or falling forward.

Now, raise your arms in front of you to about shoulder height and then lower your arms. How does that feel? Easier or harder than before? Most people feel that their arms are lighter and freer when they sit in a balanced fashion.

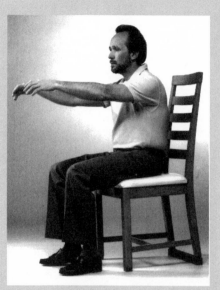

How does it feel to lift your arms when your pelvis is in different positions?

The feeling of lightness people experience when they sit well does not come from reducing the body's weight, of course. It comes from removing the interferences with natural movement. Your muscles have to fight gravity to lift your arms. If you are sitting wrong, your muscles will have to fight your own body as well to lift your arms, and the overall sensation of effort is interpreted by the body as simple heaviness. When your muscles have to do less work than ordinarily to get your arms up in the air, your body will experience this as lightness.

In the anatomically proper pelvic alignment, your back is relaxed and free, and you can raise your arms farther with less effort. This is important in typing. If your arms are not free, then your muscles will be fighting your joints and overworking to produce the movement you need. This will produce fatigue and strain.

EXPERIMENT: LATERAL AND SPIRAL STRAIN

In addition to vertical imbalance, lateral imbalance and spiral strain also create problems for computer users. Try leaning your shoulders, hips or head to one side and then raise your arms up in front of you. Notice how that sideways imbalance affects the freedom and ease with which you raise your arms forward. Or turn your head all the way to one side and notice how that spiral motion through your neck and spinal column affects the freedom and ease of your arm movements. These imbalances are often more subtle than the slump or swayback imbalances, but they create significant strain.

YOUR HANDS AND ARMS

In addition to overall body misuse, there is also strain that comes specifically from how you use your hands and arms. Some of this strain comes simply from over-tensing your muscles, and some of it comes from how you position your arms and hands.

EXPERIMENT: RELAXING YOUR ARMS AND HANDS

Take a moment to relax your belly and your breathing. Then place your hands comfortably on your lap. Let them lie still, and consciously release all the muscles in your shoulders, arms, wrists, fingers, palms, and knuckles. If you are not sure how to release the muscles, first tense them. Pick your shoulders up around your ears. Tense your arms. Tighten your hands and fingers. This will help you feel where the muscles are and what tensing is. Then cease tensing. Whatever you do to let go of tensing the muscles, do that even more. Let your shoulders settle down, let your arms rest, let your hands soften. Allow your muscles to get more and more relaxed.

Try keeping your hands gentle and soft, and now move your fingers. How lightly and fluidly can you move them? It is not necessary to make your hands tense and stiff as you move them.

Hold your hands over your thighs as though you were holding them over your keyboard. Do you hold your hands up by stiffening them or pulling your fingers back? Instead, let your hand relax into a softly curled shape. Try pressing your fingertips into your thighs as though you were typing. Do you stiffen your fingers as you press down onto the "keys"? You don't have to. Imagine you are going to press down to touch a blueberry floating in a bowl of cream just under the surface. Instead of pressing your finger down tensely onto the surface of the cream, you would gently poke down through the surface to touch the blueberry. Try "typing" that way. That will allow you to extend your fingers without tensing them.

It is important to relax your hands as much as possible while you type. If you keep your hands tense, your muscles will be stiff just at the time your fingers are being called upon to do lots of small, rapid movements. Your muscles will be fighting the movements, and this will create strain and could lead to pain and physical damage. There is a lot of time for each finger to rest in between key strokes. If you let all the fingers that are not stroking at any given instant really rest as much as possible (given that you need to hold them in position), you will find that your hands will be more relaxed and will move more freely as you type.

If you want your hands to relax, it is important not to ask them to do impossible things. If you contort your hands to stretch your fingers across the keyboard, you will certainly experience tension and strain. Instead of using one hand to simultaneously push two keys that are far apart, use two hands. Instead of reaching your little fingers sideways to push command keys, move your whole hand and arm over.

• • • • • • •

How should you position your arms and hands and, of course, your keyboard? That is a complex topic. Your hands have to face your keyboard as you type, so let's begin with an examination of the factors that determine how you orient your hands.

EXPERIMENT:
ANGLE OF PALMS AND CHEST/BACK USE

Stand up, and let your arms hang loosely at your sides. What directions do your palms face? Do they both have the same angle relative to your body?

As you stand, cave in your chest and roll your shoulders forward and toward the midline of your chest. Notice that when you do this, your palms turn to face straight back.

Try puffing up your chest, rolling your shoulders out and back, and pulling your shoulder blades in toward each other. Notice that as you do this, your palms turn to face straight in toward each other.

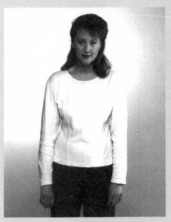

Caved in posture, palms face to the rear.

In an anatomically neutral hand position, the palms will point neither straight in toward each other nor straight back behind the body. Instead, the palms will be about halfway between those two extreme positions. Some people find that their palms point straight in or straight back when they stand as they usually do, but this is the result of some postural distortion in the chest, back, and shoulders.

Both the chest-in and the chest-out postures are very strained. Stand in a middle posture, in which your chest and shoulders are relaxed and your palms are in a half-turned position. Try pointing your palms straight in or straight back just by turning your hands. Notice that it takes muscular effort in your forearms to achieve those positions, but the half-way position is relaxed.

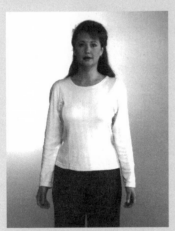

Chest puffed up, palms face inward.

EXPERIMENT: RELAXED PALM POSITION

Sit in the upright, balanced, centered position, with your arms hanging down by your side. Bend your elbows to about ninety degrees. You can imagine your hands are on a flat keyboard out in front of you. Turn your palms flat down and notice how that feels. Are you using any effort to force your palms to face the keyboard?

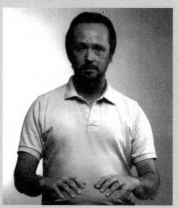

Most people will find that it takes significant muscular effort to turn their palms completely flat. Let your hands and forearms relax and notice what direction your palms move to face. Most people will find that their palms will naturally move so that they are in a half-turned position.

Keyboarding is a strenuous activity. If you keep your hands in a physically neutral position while you type, that will help reduce the effort you expend. This half-turned position of your hands is the key to comfortable hand use.

Palms half turned, wrists relaxed and straight.

EXPERIMENT: ARM HEIGHT AND ANGLE OF PALMS

Stand in an upright position with your arms by your sides and your palms in the half-turned neutral position. Raise your arms up to shoulder height in front of you. What direction do your palms face at the beginning and end of the movement?

Most people find that when their arms are at shoulder height it is natural and comfortable to hold their palms facing straight down toward the floor. Lower your arms and watch the gradual way in which your hands come back to the half-turned position. It is interesting that the anatomically natural position for the hands is flat back (pointing down) at shoulder height but half turned when the arms are down by the sides.

The way the angle of the palms relates to the height of the arms is important in keyboarding. Most people use flat keyboards (though there are dome-shaped keyboards that allow the hands to type at the half-turned angle). To type on a flat keyboard, it would seem that your hands should face flat down. However, unless your keyboard were at shoulder height, this would require extra muscular effort in your forearms and hands. Of course, putting your keyboard at shoulder height would make your neck and shoulders extremely uncomfortable.

If your keyboard is too high, your arms will have to strain to stay held up, but it will be easier to turn your palms flat. If your keyboard is too low, you won't have to hold up your arms, but you will have to expend extra muscular effort in your forearms to turn your palms flat down. What do you do?

Some people handle the problem of the palm angle by changing the position of their elbows. A simple experiment can help you evaluate this solution.

EXPERIMENT: ELBOW SPREAD AND ULNAR FLEXION

Sit up in the centered, balanced posture, with your arms hanging comfortably down by your sides. Leaving your elbows by your sides, bend your elbows and hold your hands straight out in front of you as though they were resting on a keyboard. Let your palms rest in the half-turned position. Now, move your elbows up and out to the sides, as though you were raising your wings. Notice that when you do that, your palms move into a perfectly flat-down orientation. Moving your hands into a flat-down typing position this way does orient your palms to the keyboard, but at large cost.

When your elbows are out, where does each forearm-wrist-hand unit point? Inward, as though your arms were two sides of a triangle coming to a point in front of you. However, the rows of keys lie in a straight line. If you hold your forearms on an angle, in order to position your fingers on the rows of keys, you have to bend your hands sideways toward the little finger edge of your hand. This is called *ulnar flexion*, meaning that the hand is bent toward the ulna, the bone along the little finger edge of the forearm.

Try holding your elbows high up and your forearms at about right angles to each other, so that your hands come together in a point. Then bend your hands toward the little finger edges of your hands, so that your hands now point straight ahead, as though you were going to place them on your keyboard. What does that feel like? Most people feel that pulling their little fingers out toward their forearms creates an extreme strain in their wrists. (There is a safe way to position the hands, which we will talk about shortly, when we discuss the wrists in more detail.)

There are now keyboards with the rows of keys bent into a V shape. There are also adjustable divided keyboards that can be moved into a shallower or deeper V shape. Bending the rows of keys matches the angle of the forearms to the angle of the keyboard, so the wrists don't have to be cocked outward, but it still isn't a good solution to the problem of the palm angle for most people.

Hold your elbows up and away from your sides for a while. What do you feel in your shoulders and neck? Notice that holding your elbows up creates a good deal of strain in your shoulder and neck muscles. Clearly, holding your elbows outward is not the solution to the problem of positioning your hands. Instead of using a V-shaped keyboard to compensate for a mistaken arm position, it will be better to improve the use of the whole body, shoulders and arms. (For more on this, see the section on V-Shaped Keyboards in Chapter 15.)

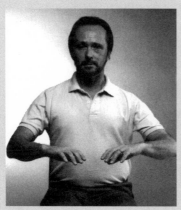

When the elbows are out, the hands point inward.

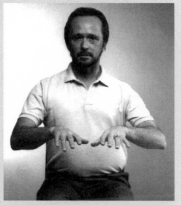

When the elbows are held out, ulnar flexion is necessary to aim the hands forward, which can produce severe wrist strain.

EXPERIMENT: ANGLE OF THE WRIST

How should you hold your wrists as you type? Sit in the centered posture, with your elbows bent so that your forearms are about horizontal and your palms somewhat turned toward each other. Hold your wrists relaxed in a fairly straight position. Now move your fingers as though you were typing. What does the movement feel like? Do your fingers move easily? Is the movement smooth or jerky?

Next, flex your wrists, that is, bend them down so your palms are brought close to the undersides of your forearms. Move your fingers as though you were typing. Notice the sensation of compression and strain. The muscles and ligaments involved in pushing your fingers down onto the keys are on the underside of the hand/wrist/ forearm unit. When your wrists are flexed, these muscles and ligaments are shortened and constricted, and the muscles and ligaments on the top of your hand and fingers are stretched taut. In this condition, your fingers cannot move freely. Notice also that when your wrists are flexed, your fingers will open and lengthen a bit, which would make it hard to position your fingers on the keys.

Try hyperextending your wrists, that is, bend them back, so the backs of your hand are brought close to the upper sides of your forearms. Move your fingers to type, and notice the feeling of tension. When your wrists are hyperextended, the muscles and ligaments are stretched and tensed, and in this condition they cannot move freely and easily. You will experience strain when you perform small, rapid, repetitive movements. Notice also that when you hyperextend your wrists, your fingers will curl up, which would make it hard to position your fingers on the keys.

When your wrists are relaxed and fairly straight (in the forward/backward direction), your fingers will be relaxed and somewhat curled, and your finger movements will be as strain-free as possible.

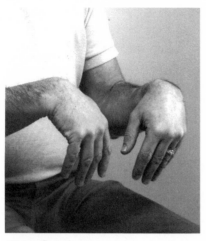

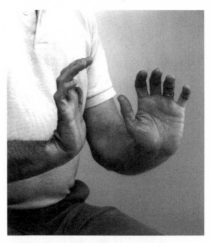

Wrists flexed.   *Wrists hyperextended.*

EXPERIMENT: ULNAR FLEXION

Ideally, to avoid the strain of ulnar flexion, your wrists should be as close to straight as possible (in the side-to-side direction) when you type. That means that the knuckle of your middle finger (counting the thumb as one of your five fingers) should line up with the middle of your forearm. However, if you are going to type on a straight keyboard, you will need to bend your wrists just a bit, and there is a safe and comfortable way to do that.

You can bend a joint by shortening one side or lengthening the other side. The image you have of what the movement should be will actually affect the movement. Rather than bending your wrist by pulling the little finger edge of your wrist tight, try gently lengthening the thumb side of your wrist just a bit. This should be such a small and gentle action that it will be almost unnoticeable. You will probably find that doing that loosens your wrist and allows you to bend it without strain. If you keep your elbows down by your sides and allow your hands to assume the half-turned position, you will not need much wrist bend at all, and bending your wrists this way will probably be comfortable for you. If it isn't, you can buy a split keyboard. (See the section on Keyboards in Chapter 15.)

So there is a solution to the problem of placing your hands on a straight, flat keyboard. A flat keyboard can be used comfortably and safely. Your elbows should be down by your sides, and your wrists should be straight, with just the slightest bit of relaxed ulnar flexion. This will allow you to use the straight rows of keys. You should hold your palms with a slight slant—your index fingers slightly higher than your little fingers. This half-turned hand position will allow a flat enough position to be comfortable on the keyboard, but the slant will be enough to take away the muscular effort needed for a perfectly flat position. (We will look at keyboard use more specifically in Chapter 15, Making Your Desktop Workstation Comfortable.)

EXPERIMENT: ARM REACH

How far in front of you should your keyboard be placed? Where should you hold your hands for greatest comfort?

Sit up in the vertical, balanced posture, with your hands in your lap and your elbows hanging down by your sides. Now imagine that your keyboard is out in front of you at about arm's length. Move your hands out to reach it. Notice that you have to raise your hands forward, up and out, and when you do this, you have to use your shoulder muscles to raise your arms. The farther you extend your arms, the more muscular effort it takes, and the longer you keep them extended, the more strain and fatigue you will feel.

Now sit with your arms hanging down by your sides. Letting your elbows continue to hang down by your sides, bend your elbows to raise your hands up in front of you so that your forearms are approximately horizontal. In that position, your shoulder muscles will be doing almost no work. ·

Of course, the muscles around your elbows will work to keep your elbows bent and your hands up. However, the weight of your forearm is considerably less than the weight of your whole arm, so less work will be necessary. In addition, since holding a weight farther from your body increases the leverage your muscles must work against, extending just your forearms means you will experience much less strain.

EXPERIMENT: ANGLE OF THE ELBOW

Sit in the centered posture, with your elbows bent so that your forearms are about horizontal and your palms somewhat turned. Hold this position for a minute or so, and notice how it feels to hold your arms this way. Now, keeping your elbows where they are, bring your hands about half way up toward your shoulders, and hold them there for a while. Notice what that feels like, and then lower your hands back to their starting position.

Most people feel that it takes more effort to hold their hands higher, and they feel their arms relax as they drop their hands down to the horizontal position again. It will be easiest to type with your wrists straight, your elbows by your sides, and your forearms approximately horizontal. Whether your arms are exactly horizontal or slightly above or below horizontal is a matter of individual comfort. Experiment with different positions and find out what is most comfortable for you.

One consideration that will have an impact on your arm position will be the orientation of your keyboard. If your keyboard slants up (meaning the edge farther away from you is higher than the closer edge), then a slight upward slant of your arms will allow you to type with your wrists straight. If your keyboard slants down, then you would want your arms slanted slightly downward to match that. (We will talk more about keyboard position in Chapter 15.)

After all these experiments in developing awareness of how the arms and hands function, we have enough information to describe the ideal arm and body functioning for typing on a computer keyboard. To find the most comfortable placement of the keyboard, first position yourself to sit comfortably. Then put the keyboard where your fingers are.

What is the most neutral, strain-free position to sit for keyboarding? That is the upright, balanced, centered position. Your elbows should hang gently by your sides and be bent about ninety degrees to bring your forearms to a horizontal position. Your wrists should be fairly straight. Your palms should be somewhat turned toward each other, and your fingers should be relaxed and curled a bit. Your keyboard should be placed so that your fingers naturally rest on the home row of keys (the ASDFG row on the ordinary keyboard). Holding your arms this way will allow you to be as relaxed as possible in typing. (See the photograph at the beginning of Chapter 15.)

There are two last elements to pay attention to in hand and arm use. One is your fingernails. If they are long, you will have to compensate for this in positioning your fingers over the keys, and you may find yourself exerting extra effort in doing this. The most natural and comfortable positioning will be possible only if your fingernails are short enough not to interfere with finger placement.

Another element is pressure and irritation. If you rest any part of your body against a hard surface, you will compress and irritate the body part that takes the pressure. This is especially true if you rest a body part against a sharp edge, since the edge will concentrate pressure over a very small area of your body. Many people rest their hands or elbows on their desks as they use a keyboard, mouse or trackball, and that can lead to irritation and injury.

EXPERIMENT: PRESSURE SPOTS

Sit at a desk or table, with your forearms out in front of you resting on the flat surface. Try moving your fingers as though you were typing. Notice the feelings of pressure in the soft under-surface of your wrist. Try resting your forearm on the edge of a book as you move your fingers, and notice how the sharp edge increases the pressure.

Type on your keyboard with your wrists resting on your desk surface. Notice that you have to hyperextend your wrists to get your fingers in position over your keyboard, which is itself a problem. And resting your wrist on your desk worsens the compression and tension in your wrist that the hyperextension causes. If you rest your wrists on the edge of your desk while hyper-extending them, there will be especially great pressure on your wrists.

Leaning your elbows on your desk as you work at your computer limits the freedom of movement at the joint, which increases stress. And of course, the simple pressure can cause irritation.

The use of the arms and hands involves a complex process of adjustment. Finding a comfortable adjustment will probably be an ongoing process of thinking about, and experimenting with, your posture and your workstation. However, when you feel your body, you will notice discomfort. Rather than letting it go on until discomfort turns into damage and damage turns into disability, you will make the changes necessary for working in comfort.

KEY POINTS

- Your arms are connected to your collar bones and shoulder blades, and are positioned largely by your spinal column/pelvis. Proper arm use begins with pelvic balance. Let your shoulders stay relaxed and down, supported on your pelvis/spinal column.
- Lateral and spiral imbalances of your hips, shoulders, or head will also create inefficiency and discomfort in your arms.
- Let your hands and arms relax while you type. Move your whole hand and arm to reach difficult keys.
- Let your hands assume a relaxed, half-turned position over your keyboard. Let your elbows fall into a relaxed position by your sides, and hold your forearms horizontal. Gently keep your wrists fairly straight, both up and down and side-to-side. If you have to bend your wrists slightly to the side, make sure to do so by opening and relaxing them.
- Don't rest your weight on your hands, wrists, or elbows. That constant pressure could lead to irritation and injury.

IMPROVING THE USE OF YOUR LEGS

Even when you are sitting, your legs are important in how you work at your computer. If your legs are tense or positioned wrong, your whole body will resonate to that discomfort, and you will be uncomfortable all over. If you use computers in a standing position, your legs are obviously a direct and crucial part of your body's support system.

RELAXATION

Simple muscular relaxation is important. Your legs have to be relaxed for the rest of your body to be relaxed.

EXPERIMENT: RELAXING YOUR FEET

The way you tense or relax your feet determines how they will touch the floor and how they will support you. Sit on a chair and take off your shoes and socks. (Are you really going to do this at the office? You should probably try this exercise where you have some privacy.)

Put your feet down on the floor, and notice how they contact the floor. How much space is there under your arch? Do you hold your toes crinkled up? Do you grip the floor with your toes? Does your right foot feel exactly like your left foot?

Pick up one foot and put it across your knee. Take hold of one toe, and pull it gently, turn it gently, roll it around gently. Then do the next toe, going on until you have done all five. Next, rub the bottom of your foot, not too hard, letting the muscles yield to the pressure of your touch and get soft.

Now put your foot down on the ground. Instead of holding your foot in its normal configuration, let it spread out to fully contact the ground. Does it feel different from before? Does it feel different from the other foot? Walk around and notice how your walk is affected by having your foot more relaxed. How does relaxing one foot affect the rest of your body? Then sit down and do your other foot. Walk around and notice how having both feet relaxed makes you feel.

Most people experience that their walk is smoother and more balanced when their feet touch the ground more fully. They realize that though they were not aware of it before, they had unconsciously been tensing their feet. They realize that created tension throughout the rest of their body, and they feel how much more comfortably they can sit or walk when they relax their feet.

EXPERIMENT: RELAXING YOUR LEGS

Sit in the centered posture. Don't press your legs together but allow some space between them. Keep your lower legs vertical, neither tucked in under you nor stretched out in front of you. Put your feet flat on the ground, and let them contact the ground. Now tighten the muscles in your lower legs and thighs. Release the muscles. Do this a few times. Then, without a preliminary tightening, release them even further, and spend a few moments concentrating gently on letting your legs hang heavily on the ground.

Pay attention to breathing softly. As you do, imagine/feel that you are gently drawing the air into your belly. Then exhale by breathing down through your legs, and out the soles of your feet into the ground. Feel the gentle flow of the air down through each part of your legs and out into the ground. Let your legs relax more and more each time you exhale. Feel how joining your breath to the ground lets your legs become relaxed and heavy.

In learning to relax your feet and legs, it is also important to pay attention to how comfortable your clothes are.

EXPERIMENT: TIGHT CLOTHES AND SHOES

Try walking around wearing loose casual clothes. Notice the rhythm and quality of your movements. Try putting on a pair of pants or a skirt that is too tight and doesn't give room for free movement. How does that make your legs feel? How does it affect your movement? What happens to your breathing? While we're at it, though this chapter is about the legs, try putting on a tight suit jacket and tie, or perhaps a turtleneck sweater with a tight neck. What does that do? Most people find that their bodies tense up to fight the restriction of the tight clothes. That creates tension and fatigue throughout the body. Ideally, your clothes should allow your body to move freely and easily.

What about your shoes? You might want to go back to the foot relaxation exercise before doing the next part of this exercise. Once your feet feel soft and comfortable, walk around barefoot, letting your feet gently mold to the floor.

Now put on your shoes and walk around. How do you feel? How does the feeling in your feet affect your overall muscle tone, posture and breathing? If you normally wear comfortable shoes, putting on shoes will probably not affect your body too much. However, if you normally wear shoes that are too tight or that don't conform to the natural shape of your feet, you may notice for the first time just how uncomfortable they are and how much tension that creates throughout your body.

If you normally wear comfortable shoes, you might want to find a pair of shoes that you know will be too tight for you. Put them on and walk around. Feel how the discomfort in your feet affects the rest of your body. Comfortable shoes are important in computer comfort.

SUPPORT

Once your legs are relaxed, it is time to examine how they function in supporting your body. It may not be obvious that your legs are part of the support system for your pelvis and spinal column and arms when you are sitting, but they are.

What is your image of the structure of your leg? Your leg attaches to your pelvis at your hip. Where is your hip? (See the picture of the skeleton in the beginning of Chapter 5.) The hip is a ball-and-socket joint, and the hip socket is at the top of your leg, surrounded by muscles. The bone by your waist that is normally called the "hip" is the lip of the pelvis (the iliac crest) and not the hip at all. Your pelvis is like a tabletop, and your legs are like the table legs. In order to sit or stand comfortably, it is important to feel how your legs/hips function as supports for your pelvis and spinal column.

If your legs are not correctly involved in your sitting posture, you will experience unnecessary strain and fatigue.

EXPERIMENT: REMOVING YOUR LEGS

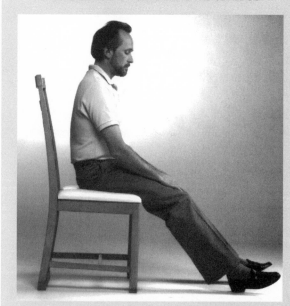

When you remove your legs, your back is not supported.

Sit in the centered posture, with your knees spread a bit apart, your lower legs vertical (neither stretched out in front of you nor tucked under you) and your feet flat on the floor. Notice the feeling of support for your posture. Now, slide your feet forward until the balls of your feet are off the floor and the weight of your legs is resting on your heels. What happens to the feeling of support for your torso? Most people immediately feel their bodies slump and the weight hang uncomfortably on their necks and backs.

Try tucking your legs back under the chair. How does that affect the feeling of support and balance for your torso? Most people feel that it takes more effort to sit upright. What do you feel in your thighs where they press against the edge of the chair? Many people find that sitting with their legs tucked cuts off the circulation and makes their legs fall asleep.

Your legs and feet are definitely an important part of overall body support. Keeping your feet flat on the floor provides important support to the rest of your body.

EXPERIMENT: KNEE–HIPS HEIGHT

Let's experiment with the relationship between the position of your hips and knees. You will need a couple of telephone books for this. Sit on a firm, flat chair in the balanced, upright position.

The height of the top surface of the seat pan should be equal to the distance between the sole of your foot (or shoe if you are wearing shoes) and the underside of your thigh. If the chair height is less than this, sit on a blanket folded to the thickness required to achieve that seat pan height. If the seat pan height is greater than this, put some books under your feet to raise the "floor." If the seat pan has a bucket or tilt back, fill it in with some towels to achieve a level sitting surface. Sit close to the front edge, without leaning onto the backrest. Notice that when you sit on the chair, your knees and hips are at about the same height.

Now, put one telephone book under your feet. Notice that raises your knees above the level of your hips. What does it do to your pelvis and low back? To exaggerate the effect, put both the telephone books under your feet. How does the movement of your pelvis affect the position of your back, chest, neck, and head?

When your knees are higher than your hips, your pelvis is rolled back, and the balance of the pelvis/spinal unit is disturbed. You wind up in a slump. Notice that position interferes with the balance of your head and increases the amount of tension you experience in your neck and shoulders and in your breathing.

Remove the telephone books, and sit with your knees and hips on the same level. Now sit on one of the telephone books. Your knees are now lower than your hips. How does that feel? How does it affect your pelvis and low back? Notice that it tends to roll your pelvis forward, creating some lordosis (concave curve) in the low back. Sit on both telephone books, and notice that increases the lordosis. Most people find that creates tension in their backs.

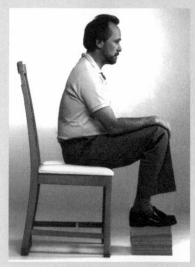

When the knees are too high, the pelvis is tipped back.

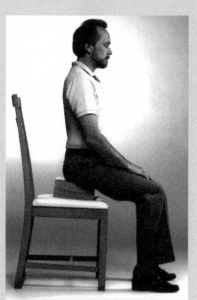

When the knees are too low, the pelvis tips too far forward.

EXPERIMENT: LEGS CROSSED

Many people sit with their legs crossed. Start by sitting up in the balanced, upright position with both your feet flat on the floor. Now put one ankle over the other knee. How does that feel? What happens to your hips, back, and neck? Try putting one knee over the other. How does this way of crossing your legs affect your body?

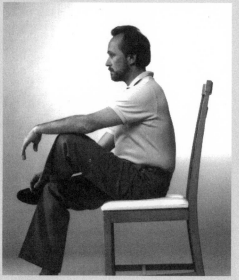

Crossing one leg over the other raises one knee higher than its hip and causes the pelvis to tip back. That rounds the lower back and makes it impossible to maintain the efficient, centered sitting posture. When I try to type with my legs crossed, my neck starts to feel a lot of strain very quickly.

Crossing the legs reduces support for the back.

Crossing your legs is fine in certain situations, but it will be very uncomfortable for computer work. Keeping your feet flat on the floor is the most efficient sitting position for keyboarding.

When you sit at your computer, both knees should be slightly lower than your hips. You will be most comfortable when your thighs slope gently down. If your knees are higher than your hips, that will rotate your pelvis backward and make it very difficult to attain and maintain the balanced, vertical sitting posture. Having your knees below your hips helps maintain the natural curves of your back. How far below your hips should your knees be? Every person is somewhat different, and I would suggest that you play with different seating arrangements until you find the exact position that makes you most comfortable. In any case, your knees won't be too far below your hips.

There are some chairs that have seat pans with pronounced forward slants. In Chapter 11, which discusses what good posture is and is not, we will examine how sitting on a very slanted seat pan affects your posture.

• • • • • • • •

Another element of leg positioning has to do with how much space you have between your legs.

EXPERIMENT: DISTANCE BETWEEN LEGS

Sit in the centered position. Press your knees and ankles together and notice what that feels like. How does it affect your low back and breathing? Notice that keeping your legs together rolls your pelvis back, rounds your back a bit, creates tension in your legs and back, and restricts your breathing.

Now spread your knees and feet about shoulder-width apart. Spreading your legs apart rolls your pelvis forward, arches your back a bit and releases your breathing—all of which creates greater relaxation and comfort.

Remember the chest-push exercise in Chapter 5? You might wish to try repeating it with your legs closed and open. Most people find that when their legs are closed, their sitting position becomes much weaker and less stable.

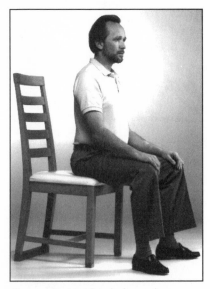

Knees apart, pelvis balanced.

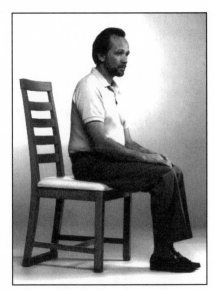

Knees closed, posture slumped.

I'm afraid sitting this way might be psychologically uncomfortable for many women. Our culture commands women to sit with their legs together. That is the ladylike way to sit, and many women feel that sitting with open knees is a man's way of sitting. Unfortunately what passes for ladylike in our culture is biomechanically false. It is weak and uncomfortable, and sitting that way makes you a pushover. So, would you rather be strong, balanced, comfortable and injury-free, or ladylike? Wearing short skirts may make it uncomfortable to open your knees, and wearing tight skirts may make it impossible to do so. You can wear pants or full, long skirts and open your knees comfortably apart.

I hold black belts in Aikido and Karate. Let me take off my computer instructor hat and put on my self-defense instructor hat for just a moment. Many women have a feeling that spreading their legs is a sexual invitation or makes them sexually available. On the contrary, using your body in a strong, free way allows you to define and protect your boundaries better. You become clearer and more assertive verbally when you are physically stronger and more balanced. And if push comes to shove, you become better able to protect yourself by running or fighting when you give up the ladylike demeanor that is supposed to keep you safe. I know that changing such a fundamental aspect of the way you present yourself can be very disturbing, but it truly is necessary to open your legs to avoid repetitive motion injuries from working at your computer.

High heels are another element of a ladylike image in our culture, but they disturb the weight placement of your feet, legs, and pelvis.

EXPERIMENT: HIGH HEELS AND FOOT FUNCTIONING

To feel how high heels affect your body as you work at your computer, you can try sitting and alternating between two different positions of your feet.

Wear flat shoes or sit without any shoes on. Where are your knees and hips? How do your ankles feel? How is your pelvis positioned, and what is your breathing like?

Now, put about three inches (seven centimeters) of books under your heels or put on a pair of tall high heels. Notice that raising your heels tips your pelvis back, taking you out of the position of easy balance. However, wearing high heels not only lifts your knees, but it simultaneously drops your toes, which adds to the sensation of leg strain. Wearing high heels as you sit creates imbalance and tension all the way through your legs and up into your hips and low back.

Once in a class I was teaching, after listening to me preach about the evils of high heels, the women got together and informed me that I was going to learn to wear high heels. They brought in a pair that fit me and coached me in how to walk in them. What an experience! I discovered that they were every bit as uncomfortable as I thought they would be. I know that there are business situations in which women (and men too) have to sacrifice how they feel to present the "right" image, but high heels should be avoided as much as possible. And when it is necessary to wear them, wear heels that are as low as possible.

• • • • • • •

In addition to relaxation and correct positioning, you also need to keep your legs moving in order to keep them comfortable. If you simply park your legs beneath you and leave them motionless as you work at your computer, the muscle blood pump (see the section on Static and Dynamic Action in Chapter 3) will not operate, and your legs could swell or become uncomfortable. In Chapter 12, on Five-Second Movement Breaks, you will learn some simple movements to make your legs more comfortable.

There is another reason why you cannot simply park your legs and ignore them. Living in your legs in an alert, vigorous and active way contributes to your ability to support your torso comfortably for long periods of sitting. Losing awareness of your legs will make it harder to sit comfortably.

EXPERIMENT: LEG/PELVIS POWER

To develop your awareness of just how your legs are related to your pelvis, try standing and pushing on a wall, with your feet far enough from the wall that your body inclines forward quite a bit. Where in your body do you feel muscles working to push? Are you pushing primarily with your arms, or do you push with your legs as well?

Try pushing by bending your knees quite a bit and then straightening your legs rapidly, as though you were trying to push the floor backward away from the wall. Notice that the shove back and down with your legs creates a strong forward shove on the wall—if you are using your pelvis correctly.

How does your pelvis connect your legs to your arms? Maintain a steady push on the wall, and gradually rotate your pelvis so that you move from tucking your tail to arching your back. What happens to the push as you do this?

Notice that when your back is arched, the force of the push shoves your shoulders back away from the wall, and when your tail is tucked, the push shoves your pelvis back away from the wall. When your pelvis is aligned properly, neither tucked nor arched, you will experience a strong push on the wall. Feeling this will give you a clear experience that your legs generate force and your pelvis transmits it to your spinal column, which in turn transmits it to your arms and hands. Many people find that this experiment transforms their awareness so that they begin experiencing the lower half of their bodies as active and powerful.

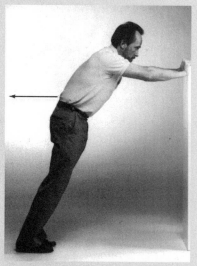

With the pelvis rotated backward, the force pushes the pelvis back.

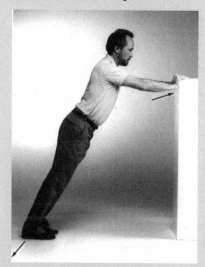

With good alignment, the force from the legs is applied to the wall.

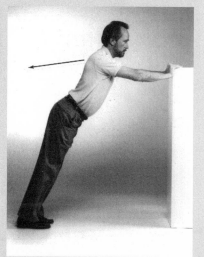

With the pelvis rotated forward, the force pushes the shoulders back

Walking with this awareness can transform the way you walk and the way you live in your legs.

PRACTICE: FEET WALKING

What is your image of walking? How do your legs and feet make your body move forward across the floor? Try walking and noticing how you walk. Do this barefoot so you can feel your feet without the interference and restriction of shoes. How do you carry your body's weight? Do you lean forward, hang behind yourself or balance yourself in the middle of your stride? Focus on your right foot as you walk. How does your foot touch the floor? Do you bang your heel into the ground or land softly? How does the weight move from your heel to your toes? How and when during your stride does your foot exert force on the floor to move you forward?

Many people feel that they swing their leg forward, and the weight of the leg drags their body forward. Some people feel that they put their foot on the floor out in front of them and then pull themselves forward with it. Some people feel that when their foot is behind them, they shove themselves forward with it. These differences are not just about how the foot is used but about the way the whole body functions.

What is the most efficient way of walking? Imagining that you are out walking shortly after a rain can provide some clues. Walk around, and try leaping over some imaginary puddles. You will have to use a long, low jump. How do you do that? Jump with your left foot forward, and notice the moment just before your right foot leaves the floor. Where is your weight, and what does your right foot do? To jump well, your weight must be forward. If you lean back, you won't get any distance in your jump. Your right leg is out behind you, your toes are bent, the ball of your foot is touching the floor. At that moment you are applying a distinct rearward shove to the floor with the ball of your foot. Your left foot is up in the air in front of you, coming down toward the ground. The rearward shove is what moves you forward.

Leaping over puddles is a somewhat exaggerated movement, but you can use the same backward push in a smaller way in ordinary walking. Try it. Keep your weight balanced between your legs—even when one is up in the air. Push back with each foot when it is behind you. This action is very similar to what you experienced in the last experiment. It is an efficient, coordinated way of using the pelvis and legs to put power into a backward thrust which will create a forward movement.

Remember your basic physics. Every action creates an equal and opposite reaction. In order to push straight backward, you would need a leg sticking out straight behind, and it could push only on walls and trees and so on. In reality, when your leg is behind you, it is on a slant, so its thrust is on a slant. You push off from the ball of your rear foot, pushing in a back and down direction. Try walking while paying attention to this process. With each step, press down and back with the ball of your back foot. Feel how the back/down energy of the foot reflects off the floor into a forward/up movement of the body. This is the most efficient way of delivering power to the ground to move you forward in a walking gait.

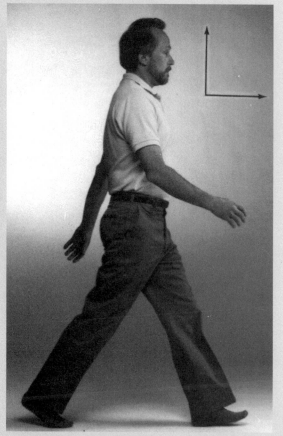

Using the legs to energize the action of walking moves the body upward and forward.

People generally experience that when they walk with this awareness of the down/back thrust of the feet, they have a ground to stand on and a foundation for themselves. The upward energy opens their posture upward. Their walk becomes more erect, clearer and more energetic. The forward energy makes them walk forward more quickly, lightly, and gracefully. When people conceive of walking as falling down onto their forward foot rather than rising off their back foot, they sag and fall down as they walk. When they pull themselves forward with the front foot, they compress and shrink. Feeling the back/down thrust leads to a way of moving that is mechanically more efficient and powerful, and it is also much more psychologically confident and alert. (See Chapter 17, Standing Computer Workstation, for more material on leg use and standing posture.)

EXPERIMENT: AIRPORT DUCK

The feeling of energizing your feet is as important in sitting as in walking.

Sit in the centered position, and notice how your feet and legs feel. Do you pay attention to them? Do you feel them? Do you live in the feeling of the contact between your feet and the floor? Or do you focus your awareness in the upper half of your body, so you can think, look at your monitor, and type?

A knickknack that I have often seen sold in airport shops is what I call an "airport duck." It is a little toy duck that sits in a bowl of water. It tips forward, puts its bill in the water, then returns to an upright position. In this exercise, you will discover what it is like to be an airport duck.

Sit in the centered position, with your legs about shoulder width apart. Lean forward as though you were going to put your nose in a bowl of water that is on a table between, and somewhat higher than, your knees. How do you do this? Do you bend in the middle of your back? Do you bend your neck?

Try doing the movement again, and this time use your hip sockets as the hinge for the movement. Remember the Pelvic Rotation and Finding Your Hip Socket experiments (in Chapter 5). Start by sitting up with your back vertical, and as you tip forward do not change the alignment of your head, neck and back. If you don't bend your back, you will experience the movement as coming from your pelvis. You will feel that your bottom will open up and project backward as you do the movement.

What happens to the weight on the soles of your feet as you bend forward? Do the movement once bending from your waist (where you wear your belt). Then keep your back aligned and move from your hip sockets. Most people feel that when they bend at the waist, very little weight gets put on their feet. But when they bend from the hips, much of the forward-moving weight goes right to their feet. Their feet and legs are active in supporting their torsos and controlling the movement, both going down and going up.

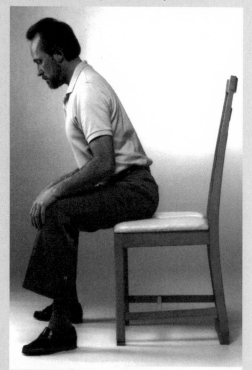

Airport Duck—Bending forward from the hip sockets, not the waist.

As an aside, the awareness of keeping your back well-aligned and moving from your hip sockets rather than your waist is important in avoiding back injuries. Though simple pressure on the intervertebral disks has not been shown to cause damage, it is well established that lifting something from a bent over and twisted position can indeed tear the disks. Imagine sitting at your desk. You drop a heavy book and bend/twist down to reach out to the side and pick it up. That lifting/twisting action is very dangerous. Keeping your back aligned and bending straight forward will do a lot to prevent injuries. This will be important later when we examine how to lift and carry a laptop computer.

EXPERIMENT: LIVELY FEET

You can become even more aware of the energy in your legs by examining the weight shift necessary for rising to a standing position. Sit on a firm, flat chair in the comfortably balanced position. Stand up and notice what movements you make to get yourself off the chair. Do you use your hands to push up? Do you use momentum to throw yourself forward and up?

Go back to the airport duck movement, and continue it even farther. As you lean forward and place your weight on your feet, keep going until you can lift your bottom a few inches off the chair. In order to do this, you have to bring your weight forward onto your legs and then use your legs to boost your body weight upward. Feel how active and alive your pelvis, hips, and legs have to be to achieve this weight shift.

Keep your whole spinal column, from your head to your tailbone, relaxed and lengthened. Hold your bottom a few inches off the chair. Now, slowly lower yourself down again, noticing the feeling of carrying and directing your weight with your legs instant by instant. Once you can move up and down comfortably just a few inches, go all the way up to standing, feeling your legs shoving downward to raise your body upward.

Keep your feet flat on the ground as you sit, and pay attention to the feeling of your feet on the floor. Pay attention to the feeling of energy in your legs and the feeling of readiness to rise to standing. You are waiting for an important and wonderful phone call. At any moment the phone might ring, and you might rise to standing to go answer it. How do your feet and legs feel? And how does that affect your sitting? If your legs are limp and unaware, they will not offer much postural support. Of course, you don't want to keep your legs tense and braced in the name of being alert and ready. Your legs should be *alive* in a calm way.

People generally experience that when they sit with a sense of how their legs contact the ground, they have a foundation for themselves. Their posture opens upward. Their pelvis and lower back will not sag. Their sitting becomes more erect, clearer, and more energetic. This new way of sitting is mechanically more efficient and powerful, and it is also much more confident and alert.

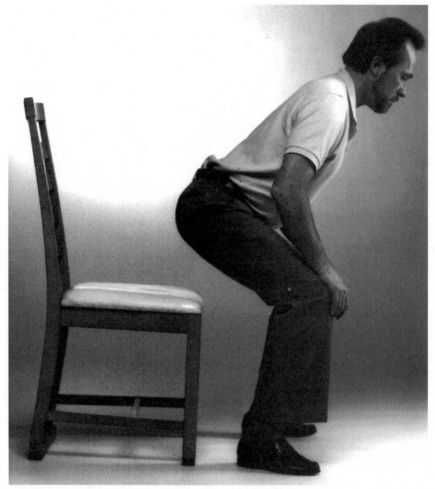

Lively feet and legs help you rise to a standing position.

EXPERIMENT: ALERT SITTING

Keeping your legs alert and lively really can make quite a difference in your mental alertness and ease. Rather than going back to the slugs-in-the-face exercise, let's try an equivalent. Have a partner sit close to you, right in your face, and shout about the benefits of eating and buying Crunchi-O's, the new improved breakfast cereal made from sun-drenched energy pellets of golden dandelion seeds. You get the idea—loud, intrusive, aggressive, and demanding.

What do you feel? How do you respond emotionally and physically to the intrusive aggression? What happens to your breathing? Does your posture change?

Sit upright in the vertical, balanced posture. Align your pelvis, soften your breathing, and open your heart. Now add the awareness of your legs. Put your legs in position, feet flat on the ground, legs spread apart, relaxed and energized. How do you feel? Does adding more awareness to your legs make you feel more whole, balanced, and strong? Have your partner shout at you again and notice how it feels this time.

Most people will feel alert and confident, ready to tell the cereal huckster to quiet down or leave. Facing impossible deadlines or impossible co-workers can be much easier if you live fully in yourself. It helps if you can stand on your own two feet and have some ground of your own to place your feet on.

If you sit and type at your computer and let your feet and legs go limp or position them so that they are not actively relating to the ground, you will find it difficult to maintain the comfortable architecture of your pelvis and spinal column. You will find that without the lively and physically balanced participation of your legs, your pelvis will not be supported. That will mean that your spinal column and shoulder girdle will not be supported, and your arms will experience unnecessary strain and fatigue. In addition, your neck and head will not be supported, and you will experience strain there as well.

Chapter 17 will be devoted to using a computer in a standing position, and proper use of the legs will obviously be crucial for that task.

KEY POINTS

- Your legs are part of the foundation and support for your whole body, even in sitting.
- Relax your feet and legs. Let your feet soften and fully touch the floor. Wear comfortable shoes.
- For best support in sitting, place your feet flat on the ground, and position your lower legs vertically. Let your knees be a bit lower than your hips, so your thighs slope gently down. Open your knees, so there is some space between your legs.
- Invest energy in your legs. Feel how your feet press your body forward and up as you walk. Be alive in your legs and feel how they support your body as you sit.
- Feeling the energy and support in your legs during stressful situations will help you become stronger, more stable and more able to handle the stress.

RELAXING AND BALANCING YOUR HEAD AND NECK

The head is last major segment of the body for us to visit on our tour of the body. Your eyes are part of your head, of course, but correct use of the eyes is such an important topic that Chapter 10 will be devoted specifically to the eyes.

Your head is supported on your pelvis/spinal column, and correct positioning of that unit provides a balanced foundation for your head. The way you move your legs and torso affects the way you move your head.

How you move your head and balance it on your spinal column also affects your whole body. Your head is a pretty heavy object, aside from all the weighty thoughts it contains. Imagine a soccer ball made out of bone and filled with oatmeal. That would approximate the weight of the head, which is about fifteen pounds for an adult.

Remember the earlier image of the torso as a flagpole being held up by guy lines on all sides? That is a good image for understanding the balance of the head as well. There are muscles along all the sides of your neck that move your head in various directions or hold it upright in position.

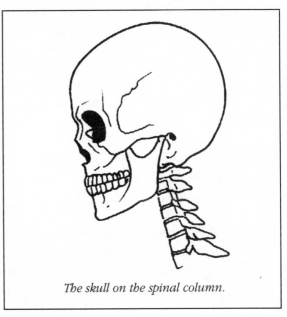

The skull on the spinal column.

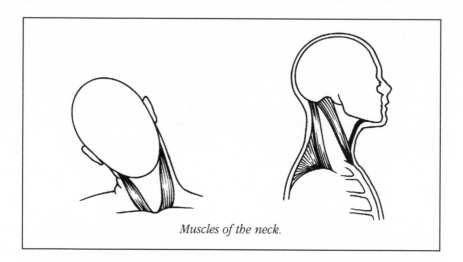

Muscles of the neck.

EXPERIMENT: HEAD IMBALANCE

It is easy to feel how the placement of your head affects your body as a whole. Sit up in the centered posture, on a firm flat chair, without leaning against the backrest. Now, tip your head over to one shoulder. Straighten it up, and repeat this movement a few times. What happens to the placement of your body when you move your head to one side?

Notice that when you hang the weight of your head off one side of your vertical support structure, you adjust your whole body. Of course, depending on how much you move and how you support yourself, these adjustments may be very small indeed. They may be so small, or you may be so unused to looking at small movements, that they could seem trivial. However, even very small weight imbalances can result in significant physical strain if they are kept up long enough.

How do you adjust your body? Some people will tip like a flagpole. They will put more weight on the sitbone on the side they shift their head to. (Remember that the sitbones are the pointy bones in your bottom that contact the chair.) Other people will bend like a bow. They will bend sideways and shift their weight to the sitbone away from the side they move their head toward. Some people will counterbalance the movement of their head with an opposite movement of their shoulders, and they will keep the weight on their sitbones essentially the same. Whichever you do, you will feel compression all the way down one or the other side of your body.

Try bending your head far forward or tilting it up and back. Notice the sensations of strain in your neck and the rest of your body. You can feel the effort it takes to maintain your sitting posture while supporting the off-center weight of your head.

Try lifting your head. What movement did you do? Most people I have worked with respond to this request by lifting their faces upward. (This way of understanding the phrase "lift your head" may be specific to speakers of American English. Some of my non-American students have responded differently.) Notice, however, that when your chin moves up, the back of your head moves down. That isn't really lifting your head. It is rotating it. Raise your chin and feel the tension in the back of your neck. How does that tension affect your whole back?

Try keeping your head still and lifting your eyes. How does that affect the muscles in the back of your neck? Most people will feel that when they look up, they automatically tense those muscles very very slightly. If you feel tension in the back of your neck as you look at your monitor, that may be a clue that your monitor is positioned too high.

The movement of lifting the face is closely related to the movement of elevating the chest that we discussed previously (in Chapter 6). People create a lot of strain and discomfort because they think that sitting up straight means puffing their chest up and "lifting their head" tall. Our culture's whole concept of "straight" is crooked. In order to use your body well, you have to get rid of the false maps of the body supplied by our culture.

There are many ways to imbalance your head. You could hold one shoulder higher than the other. You could let your head fall forward and down or off to either side. You could hold your head rotated up and pulled back. You could move your nose forward and let your head poke out, or you could pull your chin back in. And so on. When the weight of your head does not rest squarely on the spinal column, your neck will be compressed in one way or another, and your neck muscles will need to do considerable work to hold your head in position. Your neck, shoulders, and back will tense up. By finding the neutral, balanced position of your head, you will be able to relax your whole body as you sit.

EXPERIMENT: HEAD BALANCE

What is the balanced, anatomically neutral position of the head? Sit in the centered position and tip your head to the left. Now bring your head back up and continue the movement until your head is tipped to the right. When does your head cross the center line of balance so that it is no longer moving from the left toward the center but is moving from the center toward the right?

When your head is tipped over to the right, feel how the muscles on the left side of your neck work to pull your head back up to the center. And then as you cross the center and lower your head to the left, the muscles on the left side of your neck relax, and the muscles on the right side of your neck do the work of lowering your head down.

Go back and forth from left to right. Can you find the point where your head is balanced? If your head is held balanced on top of your spinal column, very little force will be necessary to keep it there. The muscles on the right and left sides of your neck will not need to work hard, and they will stay relaxed and comfortable.

Try doing this same movement sitting in front of a mirror and watching your head. Were you actually correct in identifying the balanced position of your head? Or, now that you are watching, do you notice that your head feels straight when in fact it isn't? It is informative to do a movement once on the basis of internal, kinesthetic feedback and then do it a second time with external feedback from a mirror or video monitor.

Try tipping your head back, lifting your chin way up in the air and moving your head rearward. What do you feel in your neck? Now drop your head forward, moving your chin down toward your chest. Notice the sensations this produces. Where is the point at which your head is neither forward nor backward but balanced in the middle?

Gently rotate your head up and down, as though you were nodding "yes." This is different from tipping your head. Don't move your head forward or backward. Keeping it roughly where it is, rotate your head so your chin moves up as the back of your head moves down. Feel how the muscles in the back of your neck shorten and tighten to rotate your chin up. Now move your chin down and the back of your head up.

You will not feel the muscles in the front of your neck working to bring your face/chin down (unless you press your chin down against resistance). There is a simple reason for this. Your head sits on top of your spinal column, but not the way the golden ball sits squarely on top of a flagpole. Your spinal column is not right under the middle of your head. The point of contact/support is much closer to the rear of your skull, and therefore more of your head's weight is carried forward of the contact point. Because of this, gravity pulls your chin down, and that movement doesn't take much muscular effort. In fact, you may feel the muscles on the back of your neck lowering your face down. (If you want to clearly feel the muscles in the front of your neck acting, put your hand under your chin and push up, and then force your chin down against the upward pressure.)

Rotate your head back and forth. Gradually decrease the amplitude of this movement until your head comes to rest in a neutral, relaxed position in the middle, with neither the muscles in the front of your neck nor those in the back of your neck working much. This is the natural balance position of your head. Let the muscles in your neck and shoulders relax, and let your head rest in its position of balance. How does your whole body feel when your head finds its place of balance?

When the head is balanced, the natural direction of vision is on a line about ten to fifteen degrees below the horizontal. Many people feel that their eyes are too low in this position of balance because they are used to carrying their chins too high and aiming their eyes out at the world from that position. Using your eyes in this new manner may take a bit of getting used to. (See Chapter 10 for more information on this.)

Feel the back of your head with your hands. Feel the muscles that go from your shoulders along the back of your neck and up to your skull. Feel how those muscles attach to the lower rear part of your skull. That area of the skull is call the *occiput*. Try letting your occiput float gently upward just a very slight bit. If you do the right movement, you will feel your whole spinal column all the way down to your pelvis relax and lengthen slightly upward. That sensation of freedom is a sign of the correct balance of the head on the spinal column, and it allows your whole spinal column to function in a freer more balanced way.

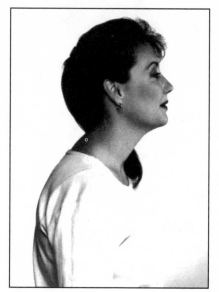
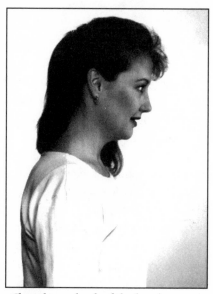

Chin up, back of the head down.   *Chin down, back of the head up.*

In addition to positioning your head for greatest ease of support, you might also pay attention to how your mouth, jaw, and face feel. Are you grinding your teeth or grimacing when you experience difficulties in your work? That won't help you bear the unbearable or accomplish the impossible. It won't even help you better accomplish what is possible. It will create tension and fatigue, which will make your job harder.

EXPERIMENT: SOFTENING YOUR FACE

It is important to relax the muscles of your face. We accumulate so much tension and unfinished emotion in those muscles. Take a moment, shut your eyes, and sit in the centered position. Feel your tongue, throat, lips and jaw. Notice how your forehead, eyelids, and cheeks feel. Are these areas of your face soft and relaxed, or are they tense? Do you hold tension in one or another part of your face?

Tense your whole face a bit. Clench your teeth. Squeeze your throat. Notice what happens in the rest of your body when you tense your face. Most people feel a stiffening and hardening throughout the rest of their bodies.

Now, let your face relax. Let your jaw relax. Soften your tongue and throat. Let your cheeks, eyelids and forehead rest. Let your mouth hang gently open a bit.

Relaxing your face is important. Not only does tension in your face communicate itself to every part of your body, but it also communicates to the people around you. If your face is tense, people pick up subliminal non-verbal messages of tension and fight-or-flight discomfort. Those messages will make them feel tense, which you will pick up. And you and the people around you will be caught in a spiraling escalation of tension and irritability. Learning to find balance and calmness is important in creating a calm and healthful work environment.

KEY POINTS

- If your head is not balanced on the top of your spinal column, the imbalanced weight and the muscular effort needed to hold it up affect your whole body.
- Let your head rest in its place of balance, which (in an upright sitting or standing position) will be at the midpoint of your head's range of movement. When your head is balanced, your eyes will aim slightly downward.
- Allow the back of your head to float gently upward, feeling that lengthening along your whole back.
- Let your jaws, throat, and face relax.

10

USING YOUR
EYES COMFORTABLY

Your eye is a wonderful mechanism. It can adjust to widely varying degrees of illumination, it can focus on objects that are very
close or very far away, and it can swivel to aim in many directions.
However, even though your eye is very adaptable, if too much adap-
tation is necessary, or if the adaptations that are necessary are mutu-
ally contradictory, eye strain will result.

Your eyes work hard when you use a computer. You may not
notice this at first, but eye strain can creep up on you. Your eyes may
feel gradually more and more uncomfortable. They may ache, or you
may experience blurred vision or difficulty in focusing. Your eyes
may be hot or irritated. Visual stress may also lead to headaches, and
eye strain will contribute to general fatigue and stress.

There are three sources of eye strain that contribute in varying
degrees to visual discomfort in computer work. Some eye strain is
due to the nature of the eye itself. Some is caused by your particular
habits of eye use, and some is caused by the way you set up your
workstation. In reducing visual discomfort, it is important to notice
how your eyes feel, track down the sources of discomfort, and then
find ways to use your eyes comfortably.

The best way to find out what is safe and comfortable for your eyes
is to ask them. They will tell you. If you don't pay attention to them
while you work, they will become more and more uncomfortable.
But if you pay attention to what you feel in your eyes, you will notice
discomforts when they are still minor, and you will be able to find
ways of reducing the discomforts.

The ways you use your eyes and the way you set up your workstation influence the positioning and use of your head and neck. A lot

of neck and shoulder strain comes from inappropriate workstation setup, and we will discuss this further in the chapters on workstation setup.

HOW YOUR EYES WORK

In order to understand how to use your eyes comfortably, it is necessary to know a bit about the structure and function of the eye. Light from objects comes into the eye through the pupil. To regulate how much light enters the eye, the iris opens in dim light or closes in bright light. The light is focused by the lens onto the retina (the inner rear surface of the eyeball). The retina receives the light and generates nerve signals to send to the brain, where they are interpreted as an image.

The eye is complex, but we can limit our discussion to the factors that influence your visual comfort at the computer. The key factors in visual comfort are: lubrication of the eye surface, focusing of the eyes, aiming of the eyes, object clarity, lighting, and general fatigue and stress.

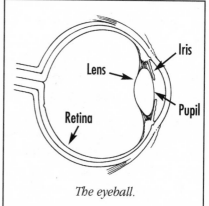

The eyeball.

LUBRICATION

The eyes produce a film of tears to cover the cornea (the outer surface of the eye). This film supplies oxygen and nutrients to the cornea and also lubricates it. As we age, the film thickens and becomes less efficient. Noxious fumes, especially smoke, and dry or dusty air, as well as various drugs can interfere with the functioning of the tears. The quality of office air is important in eye comfort, and if your eyes are uncomfortable at work, you may wish to do some reading on this topic.

When the functioning of the tears is interfered with, the surface of the cornea can become irritated and itch, and your vision can become blurred. Rubbing your eyes to relieve the itch is a natural response, but it will irritate them further.

When you use computers or read, it is especially important to keep your eyes well-lubricated. Blinking spreads the tears over your eye, so it is important to blink often. Don't get so involved staring at your screen that you forget to blink. If blinking doesn't help, you may wish to consult an ophthalmologist.

FOCUSING

Rays of light from objects at various distances need to be focused onto the retinal surface, and this is done by changing the shape of the lens. The lens is essentially the same shape as a magnifying glass, convex on both sides, and it is attached all around its edge to a band of muscles, the ciliary muscles. The lens is elastic. In order to focus on near objects, the ciliary muscles contract and make the lens rounder. In order to focus on distant objects, the ciliary muscles relax and the lens becomes flatter. The point to keep in mind is that it takes *work* to focus on near objects.

In complete darkness, when the eyes are resting, the natural shape of the lens leads to a visual focus distance of around thirty-two inches (eighty centimeters). Focusing on an object closer than that requires some work to reshape the lens, and the nearer it is, the more work it takes. However, it is not just the object distance that determines how much work it takes for the eyes to focus. The elasticity of the lens decreases with age, and so as people get older, it takes more work to reshape the lens and focus on close objects.

The near point of visual focus is the nearest distance at which an object can be brought into clear focus. The near point is determined by how strong the focusing muscles are and how elastic the lens is. In someone who is forty years old, the near point can be around seven inches (eighteen centimeters), but by sixty it could be around thirty-eight inches (one hundred centimeters). After about forty, the speed and precision of eye focusing lessen as well.

Fatigue is also a factor in close focus. In prolonged close work, the muscles act continuously to focus the lens, and they fatigue. The eye muscles, after all, are muscles like any others, and the same rules about static holding and fatigue apply to them as to any other muscles. As the muscles tire, they lose their ability to pull the lens into shape, and it becomes harder to focus on close objects. The lens itself is affected by prolonged close focus. It may maintain the close focus shape for a time, and that will make refocusing on more distant objects harder.

EXPERIMENT:
FOCAL DISTANCE AND MUSCLE STRAIN

Hold up a pencil in front of you at arm's length and focus on the eraser. Gradually bring the pencil closer to your eyes, keeping your eyes focused on the eraser. Make sure to keep blinking at a normal rate. If you don't, your eyes will become uncomfortable.

Notice the sensations as the pencil comes closer and closer to your eyes. At what distance can you no longer focus clearly? Move the pencil slightly closer, and try to force your eyes to bring the pencil back into focus. What do you feel? That sensation is the sensation of muscular strain.

Just so you won't be left with a feeling of strain, shut your eyes for a moment and cover them gently with the palms of your hands. Don't rub your eyes, as that may irritate them. Let your eyes relax. Take a deep breath, let it out, and as you do, let the muscles in and around your eyes soften and relax.

Sit in the centered position. Put something—a cup or a stapler or whatever—on a shelf a bit below your eye level. Sit about forty inches (about one hundred centimeters) away and gradually move your chair closer. At what distance do your eyes feel the least strain in focusing on the cup? What do you feel in your eyes and face when you move closer than this? The distance at which you feel the least strain is the right distance for your monitor. As a general rule, that distance will be about an arm's length or a bit more.

Comfort is a continuing quest. During my work on the second draft of this book, while I was polishing the preceding paragraph on monitor distance, I was simultaneously writing about monitor distance and examining what I was feeling in my eyes as I looked at my screen. And I discovered that I felt more comfortable if I moved the monitor back another three inches (about seven centimeters). Do we ever arrive at static perfection? Not as far as I can tell. We keep changing, our work keeps changing, and we have to stay alert to what we need at each moment to be most comfortable.

AIMING

Muscles inside the eyeball focus the eye on objects. Muscles outside the eyeball roll the eye around in the socket to aim it at the various objects we look at.

There are six muscles around the eyeball. Think of the eye as a beach ball with ropes taped to its circumference. You can also imagine that the beach ball has a circle painted on its front to represent the pupil. You are standing behind the beach ball with the ropes held in your hands. If you pull on the rope attached to the top of the ball, it will roll back and the pupil will aim upward. If you pull on the rope attached to the right side, the ball will turn to the right in a

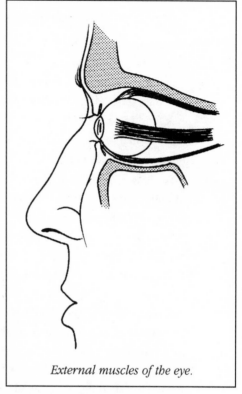

External muscles of the eye.

clockwise motion. And so on. The six muscles of the eye act in combination to create movement in any of the directions we can look.

A computer user spends time moving his or her eyes left and right across lines of text on the screen, as well as up and down from line to line on the screen and from the screen to objects on the desk. All of this takes work. In addition to moving your eyes, the ocular muscles serve to stop the movement of your eyes. They will keep your eyes fixed in position when you want to keep looking at just one thing. Computer users can spend a lot of time staring fixedly at the screen, and this is another example of static holding. (Actually, even when you stare at the screen, you will still be moving your eyes a bit, but maintaining a fixed stare is close enough to a static use of the eyes to count.) Both static holding and the work of moving your eyes can create fatigue and eye strain.

EXPERIMENT: THE EFFORT OF MOVING AND HOLDING

It is important to be able to notice and identify the sensations of muscular strain in your eyes. Sit about three feet from a wall and draw an imaginary line from your nose to the wall. The point on the wall where the line touches will serve as the center of your visual field. Pick four points around the center point to move your gaze to—one point about a foot to the left, one about a foot to the right, one about a foot up, and one about a foot down.

Now this is important! You are working at a nuclear power plant, and one of the main pipelines has ruptured. If you don't manage to watch the dials, the whole thing will blow up, and you will become nothing but a radioactive smudge on the horizon. Move your eyes back and forth from the left point to the right, fast, with anxiety and effort. Feel your eye muscles working. Notice the feelings in your eyes. Now move your eyes up and down, from point to point. Again, feel the strain in your eyes. This time, of course, you will feel the strain in a different set of muscles. (You may also notice that the muscles in your neck respond to each change in the direction of your gaze.)

The dial in the middle is the most crucial one. Look at the point in the middle. Hold that point tightly with your eyes. This is the sensation of static strain in your eyes. Do you stare at your screen this way?

Your eyes have to do a lot of movement to move across a page of text on your screen, and fatigue affects how your eyes move to aim at the text. The field of clearest vision, which is used for reading and other fine detail visual tasks, is a small circle in the center of the visual field. It is about half an inch across (about one and a quarter centimeters) at a normal reading distance. In order to get a clear image of a line of text, the eye scans the line in a series of jumps, taking in a piece of the line at each stopping point. When the eye muscles are fatigued, they cannot move the eye precisely and double vision can occur. If you keep working and try to force your eyes to focus, that will cause even more fatigue.

Sitting too close to your screen not only fatigues the eye by making it harder to reshape the lens, but it also forces the eye to do more work to scan material. When you are close to something you are looking at, the area taken in by the circle of visual clarity is small. You have to move your eyes a greater number of times to take in the whole object. Sitting farther away, the same visual angle takes in more area, and so your eyes are not required to do as much work in looking at an object.

OBJECT CLARITY

In close work, such as reading, it will require less work from the eye to focus the image when the object is at a greater distance. However, at a greater distance, fine details lose their clarity, and trying to focus on fine details when they are not clear is also a source of visual fatigue.

How clear an object is depends on a number of factors, among them, size, visual form, contrast, and illumination. If the material you are looking at is very small, you will bring it closer to you to see the fine detail. If the visual form is complex, it will take more effort to recognize and understand it. If there is good contrast between the object you are looking at and its background, that will make it easier to see. However, some contrasts make it harder to see, as, for example, looking at a bright red object on a bright blue background. Looking at both red and blue, the eye has to adapt to long and short wavelengths of light simultaneously, which it cannot easily do.

EXPERIMENT: OBJECT CLARITY

Sit far back from your computer, perhaps forty inches (one hundred centimeters) or at least an arm's length. At that distance, the clarity of what you are looking at on the screen will be a major factor in how comfortable your eyes will be.

Type a paragraph of text, and duplicate it a number of times. Change two of the paragraphs to a very small point size, and then change one of those to bold face. Which is more comfortable to read? Change another paragraph to a large point size. How does that affect readability?

Display the paragraph in different fonts. Do different fonts feel more or less comfortable to read? Try adjusting the monitor to provide very poor contrast between the text and the background. How do your eyes feel then?

What your eyes *feel* as they read the different paragraphs is your best evidence for the right way to set up your computer.

Some computers or task setups may not allow you to change fonts, font sizes, etc. to achieve a visually comfortable work situation. If your current setup is not visually comfortable, is there any way to create changes? If not, you will need to be especially careful to take rest breaks and look away from your computer frequently.

LIGHTING

Lighting involves a number of complex interactions in the eyes. The eye can adapt itself to the very dim light of a candle and the very bright light of the sun. When illumination is low, the retina increases its sensitivity and the pupil dilates to admit more light. When illumination is high, the retina decreases its sensitivity and the pupil constricts. However, the eye cannot adjust to both low and high levels of illumination simultaneously, and it cannot easily adapt to constantly changing levels of illumination. If illumination levels keep changing, the retina may not be able to adapt fast enough, and the muscles that control pupil size will fatigue.

When you are using your computer, your visual field should contain only objects of approximately the same brightness. If your visual focus is on a relatively dim object, but your visual field also contains spots of bright light, the eye will adapt to the bright spots and you will not be able to see the dim object well. The computer screen is actually a fairly dim object, and it can easily be outshined by electric lights or by windows admitting either diffuse daylight or direct sunshine.

Even if you don't simultaneously see bright and dim objects, you may be looking back and forth from a dim screen to a brightly lit book. In that situation, your pupils will still have to keep shifting back and forth between opening and closing. The muscles that control the dilation or constriction of your pupil will be working constantly, and that will fatigue them.

In addition to relative brightness of different objects, the absolute amount of light in your visual field is also important. The pupil adapts to low levels of illumination by increasing its size. When the pupil becomes larger, light rays pass through the edges of the lens, which produces some scattering of the light, and the visual image is not focused on the retina as well. In brighter light, when the pupil becomes smaller, light rays pass primarily through the center of the lens, and the visual image is focused on the retina better. So in bright light visual acuity improves.

We have a situation with some conflicting requirements for visual comfort. Brighter images allow better focusing, but the computer monitor is relatively dim. In low illumination, speed and precision of eye focus are reduced, and the near point of focus moves farther out. However, in low illumination, the tendency is to bring objects closer so they occupy a larger portion of our visual field and we can see them better. So with lower illumination, the muscular work necessary to focus on near objects increases, while at the same time we tend to bring things closer.

To make matters worse, with increasing age, higher illumination is needed in reading. At age fifty, one-and-a-half times more illumination is needed than at age twenty-five, and by sixty-five over two-and-a-half times the amount is needed. Yet the computer screen stays fairly dim.

How can you adjust all these competing factors?

EXPERIMENT: ILLUMINATION

Sit about an arm's length from your computer. Call up onscreen a paragraph of text to read, and have a book in front of you as well. Now, spend some time experimenting with different levels of illumination in the room and different levels of brightness on your screen or on the book.

What is it like to turn your screen up to maximum brightness and your general illumination down low? What do your eyes feel if your screen is dim and you position a desk light to illuminate your book very brightly? How far should the screen and the book be from you? Which screen fonts should you use at which distances and which levels of illumination? There are so many combinations of conditions that it would be hard to enumerate them all. However, if you maintain an inquiring attitude and pay attention to the sensations of comfort or discomfort in your eyes, you can continue to experiment with your work conditions and eventually find what is most visually comfortable for you.

Glare is an extreme lighting condition. Glare is the painful experience of having your eye overloaded by light. If a light is very bright, you will experience discomfort if you look directly into it, and your eyes will not be able to adapt to it and reduce the discomfort. On the other hand, a light source can be uncomfortable not because of its absolute level of brightness but because it is much brighter than what your eyes have adapted to. You have experienced this when stepping out of dim movie theater into a bright sunny afternoon.

EXPERIMENT: GLARE

Though we have all experienced glare in one situation or another, very few of us have paid attention to the experience of glare. Pick up something to read or call up some text on your computer. Position a light so that it shines directly into your eyes as you read, and notice the sensation. What do your eyes do to try to handle the glare? What happens in your facial muscles?

Notice also the effort it takes to compete with the glare and focus on the text you wish to read. How is it that many people work day after day in a work situation that is visually uncomfortable and yet either don't think about it or don't do anything about it? Pain is a message from your body that things need to be better!

FATIGUE AND STRESS

One last element of visual comfort is your overall comfort level. If you are generally fatigued or stressed out, that will affect your eyes. An experiment you might not wish to try would be to stay awake for a couple of days preparing your tax forms on your computer and then see how your eyes feel. Whatever visual strain you may experience from any of the other sources described in this chapter, general fatigue and stress will exacerbate the strain.

EXPERIMENT: FEELINGS AND VISION

All your muscles respond to your thoughts and feelings, and your eye muscles are no exception. Imagine that you are looking at something scary and painful, perhaps a horrible car crash with bleeding victims lying on the road. Notice how your eyes feel. Now imagine that you are looking at a peaceful and pleasant country scene. What changes?

Most people feel that their eyes tense up when they imagine a painful scene and relax and get more comfortable when they think of something pleasant. If your work involves a lot of emotional pressure, you will undoubtedly feel tension in your eyes as you look at your monitor or paper documents.

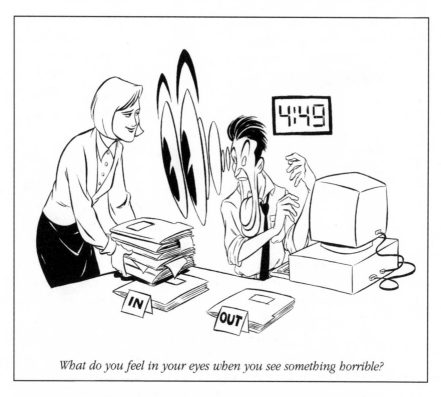

What do you feel in your eyes when you see something horrible?

Another element that affects your vision is the aesthetics of your surroundings. If you pay attention, you will feel how your eyes respond to ugliness and beauty. It isn't just our souls that respond to beauty, but all of us. Both a beautiful sunset and an elegant workplace induce feelings of comfort and relaxation in us.

COMFORTABLE EYES

After talking about the sources of visual stress and experimenting with feeling the sensations of visual stress, it is time we moved on to the topic of visual comfort.

The first thing to think about regarding eye problems is glasses. Have you had your eyes checked by an ophthalmologist, a physician who specializes in eye care? Are your eyes healthy? Is your vision adequate or do you need glasses to correct your vision? Computer work is visually stressful enough without the added stress of eye disease and uncorrected vision.

If you are using bifocals, pay attention to how they feel. Are the focal distances of the bifocals correct for computer work? Bifocals are usually designed for two distances—ordinary reading which is about twelve inches (thirty centimeters) and distance vision which is beyond twenty feet (about six meters). The monitor should be at about arm's length or a bit more for greatest comfort, which is farther than the near focus of bifocal glasses and much nearer than the far focus. You may need special computer bifocals or even trifocals designed to allow focus on both paper material and the monitor.

In addition to the focal distance, it is also important to notice the head position your bifocals require. Do you have to cock your head back or drop your head forward to see your work out of the appropriate area of the glasses? If so, you will wind up with considerable strain. You may need to have bifocals designed specifically to allow you to look at the particular elements of your workstation that you have to work with. The bifocals should allow you to keep your head in its position of balance (see Chapter 9) and move your eyes to focus on your monitor or paper documents.

• • • • • • •

Resting and relaxing your eyes is very important in avoiding fatigue and maintaining comfort. The following experiments and practices will help you feel what it means to rest and relax your eyes. You will be able to use the practices on an ongoing basis to help keep your eyes comfortable in your daily work.

PRACTICE: PALMING YOUR EYES

A commonly recommended way to rest your eyes is called *palming*. Shut your eyes. Rub your hands together, not vigorously but with a soft and smooth movement. Let your hands relax and soften. Then put your palms over your eyes and hold them there for a minute or so. Let your eyes enjoy resting in the warmth and darkness of your hands. Let your eyes become as soft and relaxed as your hands. Make sure not to press on or rub your eyes, since that could irritate them.

An alternative to palming your eyes is to close your eyes and cover them with a cool, damp cloth. You may find this more soothing than warmth, especially if your eyes are hot or sore.

PRACTICE: RELAXING YOUR EYES

You can also learn to keep your eyes relaxed even while you move and use them. Sit in the centered position and shut your eyes. Without moving your head, move your eyes to look up, down, right, and left. What do you feel in your eyes? Are you exerting *effort* to look in the different directions? Try letting the movements of your eyes be soft and fluid. Move your eyes slowly and gently. It will help if you don't move too far in any direction. Moving your eyes all the way to the edge of their range of motion takes more effort than staying in the middle.

Start moving your eyes in gentle, soft, smooth, curvy lines. Make sure to let your forehead, cheeks, mouth, and tongue relax as you move your eyes. Try some circles and figure eights. Feel how your eye muscles work to move your eyes. Is there some particular spot in the movement that is tense or hesitant? Let the places where you feel any strain soften and release.

Once you are moving your eyes in this relaxed way, slowly and gradually open them—*and don't grab the world with your eyes*. Let your eyes look at the world softly, as though it's not really important that they see anything clearly. You will probably find that you can see just as much, just as well, but with more ease and comfort.

PRACTICE: SOFT EYES

Normally we concentrate our awareness in the center of our visual field. *Soft* eyes is the skill of using central and peripheral vision in a more equal way to pay attention to more of the environment than our normal tunnel vision does. This way of using the eyes comes from the martial arts, where it is used to scan the environment and attend to numbers of people attacking all at once. Soft eyes is useful more for picking up movements than fine details, but it is a relaxing way to see and is worth practicing just for that reason. You may not want to use soft eyes when you are focusing specifically on your computer monitor, but it will help you rest your eyes during breaks from computer work.

Pick a distant spot to focus your eyes on, and keep looking gently at that spot. Make sure to keep blinking at a normal rate. Without moving your eyes, pay attention to what is already in the left side of your peripheral visual field. Now notice the right side. Now the top, and now the bottom. Blink occasionally. Now pay attention to the whole of your visual field, gently, without gripping the world with your eyes. Most people experience this as a soft, embracing, and relaxing way to use their eyes.

PRACTICE: REFOCUSING YOUR EYES

You can also learn how to focus your eyes with less effort. Sit in the centered position and close one eye, or cover it with your palm. Hold up one arm in front of your face and raise one finger. Now focus your open eye first on the tip of that finger and then on a point far off in the distance. What do you feel in your open eye? Do you feel any tension or effort in moving your eye? Do you feel any tension in the eye you have closed? Try your other eye. Does it feel different? In what way?

Close both your eyes, and put one hand gently over them. Without straining the muscles in your eyes, slowly move your visual focus back and forth between close and far away. Can you allow your eyes to feel soft and loose as you do this? Relax your mouth, your cheeks, your forehead and your eyelids as you focus your eyes.

The positioning of your head also affects the level of tension or relaxation in your eyes.

EXPERIMENT: HEAD AND EYES

Call up some text on your monitor. Try lifting your chin way up in the air so that you have to aim your eyes out past the lower edges of your eye sockets. What do you feel in your eyes?

Now put your chin down toward your chest and read your screen by looking out past the upper edges of your eye sockets. Notice the sensations this produces.

When your head is at an extreme angle, the muscles in your eyes have to work hard to aim your eyes at the screen, and you can feel this in the sensation of muscular strain. When you look ahead with your head and eyes in a neutral, balanced position (as described in Chapter 9), your eyes will do much less work, and they will feel much more comfortable.

In an upright and balanced position, the natural line of vision for our eyes is on a line about ten to fifteen degrees below the horizontal. Many people find it so unfamiliar to let their eyes rest in this line of sight that even when it feels physically right they still have the sense that it can't be right. In this position, people who are used to looking up will feel that they are looking down. It is true that they are looking more downward than they are used to, but it is just down enough to be most relaxed and balanced. The only way to get more comfortable with this new position is to persist with it until it comes to feel right.

If you take care to *feel* your eyes as you work at your computer, you will know what workstation set up makes your eyes most comfortable. If you relax your eyes as you use them and take regular rest breaks (see Chapters 12 and 14), you will be able to work in much greater comfort.

KEY POINTS

- Some eye strain is due to the nature of the eye, some to your habits of eye use, and some to your workstation setup.

- Keep your eyes well-lubricated by blinking enough. Don't rub your eyes when they are uncomfortable.

- Close focus requires extra work. Place your monitor an arm's length or a bit more from you.

- Don't overwork and fatigue your eyes. Take rest breaks, do eye relaxation and movement exercises, and look off into the distance periodically.

- Find a level and manner of lighting that illuminates paper documents enough to make reading them easy yet doesn't overpower the screen or create glare on it.

- Harmonious surroundings and feelings will produce a sense of relaxation in your eyes.

- Have your eyes examined and make sure to obtain glasses that are adapted to the specific requirements of your computer use.

11

WHAT GOOD SITTING POSTURE IS AND IS NOT

In this chapter, I'd like to take a moment to compare the centered sitting posture with other commonly recommended styles of sitting. The more you understand about the thinking underlying the various methods of sitting, the better you will understand why I recommend the centered style of sitting.

MUSCLE WORK AND DISK PRESSURE

Researchers trying to determine the optimal sitting posture for computer use have focused on two elements: muscle work and intervertebral disk pressure. Muscle work is just what it sounds like, the amount of work your muscles have to do to keep you in a given position. Different positions can take more or less work to maintain. For example, when you stand up, the weight of your torso is supported by the bones of your legs, and so your back muscles do relatively little work. But if you bend over forward, your back muscles then have to hold up much of the weight of your torso. If you lean back against a wall, the wall and your legs share the weight, so your back does little work and your legs do even less than in ordinary standing.

The optimal sitting posture would have the lowest general levels of muscle work and would make the greatest use of the larger, stronger muscles rather than overworking smaller, weaker muscles. There is a trade-off between work done by different sets of muscles as you sit and work at the computer. When you slump and let your torso hang on your bones and ligaments, the muscles that ordinarily hold up your torso do less work because they aren't holding you up. However, since your arms and head are not supported well by the spinal column and pelvis, the muscles that support your arms and head have to work harder (as you experienced in Chapters 7 and 9). (Not only that, but hanging on your ligaments imposes uncomfortable and damaging strain on parts of your body that were not designed for this.)

Intervertebral disk pressure is the amount of pressure on the cartilage disks that separate the vertebrae. Some research has suggested that high levels of pressure on the disks damage them and that reducing pressure leads to the reduction of back injuries. There has been much debate about this theory, but there is no definitive evidence that the pressures encountered in sitting lead to injury or that reduction of disk pressure actually reduces back strain or injury. Some of the research on sitting has focused on the attainment of a sitting posture that would reduce pressure on the disks, but this may or may not turn out to be of importance.

There is a trade-off between how much work you do with your muscles and how much pressure you put on your disks. When you slump, your muscles do less work because they aren't working to hold you up. However, in that bent over posture, the vertebral column bends, and this compresses the intervertebral disks. When you sit up, there is less pressure on the disks, but your muscles have to work harder. Researchers have tried to find sitting positions that reduce the compression of the disks while not increasing the workload on the muscles. Given the lack of evidence that the pressure on the disks is harmful, this may not be important, but it has been a significant factor in the thinking behind some recommendations for appropriate sitting posture.

Unvarying levels of pressure on the vertebral disks reduce the diffusion of interstitial fluid into the disks, which reduces available oxygen and nutrients as well as waste removal. (See the discussion on static holding in Chapter 3.) Good posture is not a tense, static position. Good posture is a dynamic process in which the body continuously sways around a central line of balance. The optimal sitting posture would allow and encourage movement, which will produce variations in the pressure on the disks and aid in diffusion of fluid into and out of them (as well as aiding in blood flow through the muscles).

SITTING STYLES

There are two different styles of sitting posture that have commonly been recommended for computer users. I call them the *straight up* and the *reclining* styles of sitting. There is a third style sometimes recommended, and I would call it *half-standing*. The term I use for the sitting posture I recommend is *centered*.

The straight up style is just what it sounds like. Many illustrations of good computer sitting posture show a person sitting in a very straight posture, with ninety degree angles at the knees and hips and with the legs close together. The straight up posture demands more muscle effort than slumping does, but it reduces the pressure on the disks.

The straight up and centered styles are superficially similar. The key difference is that in the centered style the relaxed balancing of the pelvis is the foundation for the positioning of the torso. In the straight up style, the muscles of the back pull the body up into position.

The straight up style is a very *elevated* way of sitting. Invariably, in illustrations of the straight up style, the chest is elevated and the body is carried high. Of course, when the chest is elevated, the back is compressed and pulled down. Perhaps this has been accepted because people focus so much on the front of the body, on putting on a good face, and they don't really feel the three-dimensional fullness of the body and its rear.

This elevated body position is so deeply embedded in our culture's ideal

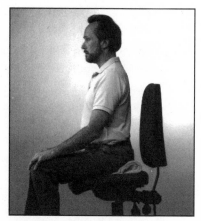

Centered sitting posture.

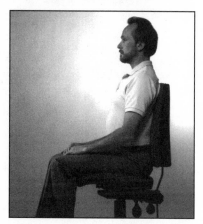

Straight up sitting posture.

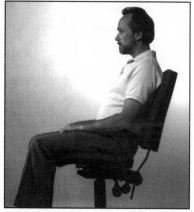

Reclining sitting posture.

of good posture that nobody even notices or comments on the idea of lifting the body. Without the contrast provided by the centered style of sitting, the upward-lifting element of the straight up style is invisible. You can see the same upward orientation in ballet, gymnastics, and often in fashion modeling. The idea behind this upward orientation is the appearance of elongation, lightness, elegance, dignity. It is interesting how often we describe goodness or value in terms of upward orientation and height—consider a lofty ideal, a superior product, or a high grade.

However, hardly anyone will really sit in the straight up posture and almost never for any length of time. There is a simple reason for that: it hurts to sit that way. It uses the muscles of the back to rotate the pelvis and pull the torso into position, and those muscles just aren't designed for that job. Most people recognize the pain caused by the straight up style, and they won't sit that way even if they believe it is the best way to sit.

Another element of the straight up style also adds to the effort required of the back muscles. Sitting with a ninety degree angle between the thighs and torso puts the body into an L shape and places most of the body's weight near the rear edge of the base of support. Leaning even just a bit back from the balanced position of the pelvis makes it impossible to anchor the body's weight in the hip sockets. It creates a posture that is tense and unstable, and it interferes with breathing and mobility (see Chapter 5). To reduce the effort that it takes to sit up when the weight is too far back, the straight up style uses a backrest to help support the body's weight. However, this encourages people to lean back, which perpetuates the problem and the need for a backrest.

The use of a backrest is also based on the idea that pressing the spinal column forward with a lumbar support will help maintain the normal curves of the spinal column and thereby decrease pressure on the disks. However, the straight up approach confuses cause and effect. Aligning the pelvis correctly will position the spinal column properly, but pressing the spinal column forward with a lumbar support will not align the pelvis correctly. Using a backrest to maintain proper back alignment distracts people from feeling proper pelvic functioning and perpetuates the need for the backrest.

Two other aspects of the straight up style also contribute to its effortfullness. Keeping the knees close together increases the effort expended by muscles in the back and torso (see Chapter 8). And last-ly, the muscular tension in the back leads to a bracing of the whole body, which is an overall state of static holding.

The centered sitting style encourages the body to support its own weight efficiently and elegantly, as it is designed to do. In centered sit-ting, the backrest is not necessary (though it can be used for an occa-sional change of position). In contrast to the straight up style, the cen-tered style of sitting uses the psoas and iliacus to create proper pelvic alignment and does not overwork the back muscles. The psoas and ili-acus are designed to bring the body to an erect position and do not get overworked by this movement. With the use of the towel roll for pelvic support, the psoas and iliacus aren't even required to do the full amount of work necessary to maintain an upright posture. Spreading the legs is also important because it arches the back a bit, which helps to reduce the amount of work needed to hold the back in position.

In addition, the centered style of sitting leans the body slightly for-ward into something of a pyramid shape, a posture that moves the body weight forward from the rear edge of the base of the support and that is therefore more stable and relaxed. And rather than keeping the body in a tense, static position, the centered style of posture places the body in a state of relaxed balance that allows movement. The centered style features an erect posture, which results in less disk compression, it avoids the inappropriate use of the back muscles usually required for erect posture, and it encourages continuing movement.

The muscular effort exerted by the arms is also a factor in com-puter use. When your elbows hang close to your sides, your arm muscles exert less effort in keyboarding. Your arms are in much the same position in both the straight up and the centered positions. However, in the straight up posture, the tension in the back and neck spreads to increase the tension and effort expended by the arms. So in this respect too the centered posture is more efficient.

• • • • • • •

In an effort to avoid the strain associated with the straight up style, many people have moved toward the equally inappropriate reclining style. People who recommend this sitting posture believe that lean-ing back onto a backrest offers the most stable and comfortable sit-ting posture. The argument is that leaning back onto a backrest allows the chair to support much of the weight of the torso so that the muscles can relax. In addition, a pad is used to press the vertebrae in the lower back (the lumbar area) forward to approximate the natural curve of the low back. This avoids the backward rotation of the pelvis and the rounding of the back that leaning back would cause, and it therefore relieves pressure on the disks.

The problem with the reclining style is that it significantly distorts breathing and the use of the head/neck unit and the arms. When you incline your torso toward the rear, you do not let your head tip back as well. In order to look at your monitor, you have to keep your eyes horizontal or somewhat below the horizon. If your torso leans back, in order to compensate, your head must lean forward and down. This movement compresses your chest and interferes with your breathing. And when your head is held forward rather than balanced atop your spinal column, your neck muscles have to work harder to hold it up.

In addition, when you lean back with your torso, you have to reach out forward with your arms to get to the keyboard. Instead of letting your elbows hang down by your side, you have to keep them held out forward, which is very fatiguing. Some people try to deal with this by using arm rests on the chair or wrist supports by the keyboard, but that too is problematic. (See the sections on wrists and chairs in Chapter 15.) It freezes people into a single position and further decreases opportunities for large movements. It requires that all the effort and movement of typing be done by the hand and wrist rather than the arm as a whole, and in addition it puts continuous pressure on the body part touching the support.

A third effect of the reclining style is to cultivate a limp, dissociated sense of the body. Your body is an elegant, powerful machine, fully capable of supporting itself when used well. Leaning back, reducing awareness of the floor and your legs, reducing awareness of the body's power to support itself—this puts you into almost an hypnotic state of loss of body contact.

A fourth negative effect of the reclining style is to reduce overall body movement. It is harder to move around when you give your weight over to the chair and cave in your torso. That in turn reduces the pumping action that helps blood flow through the muscles and helps fluid diffuse in and out of the vertebral disks.

What the reclining style gains in reduction of muscular effort in the torso and reduction of intervertebral disk pressure, it loses in increased effort in the arms and neck, and reduction of breath, movement, and body awareness.

A third style of computer sitting sometimes recommended is the *half-standing* style. In this style, the seat pan of the chair is tilted forward a fair amount. (See the section on chairs in Chapter 15 for further discussion.) This sitting posture is midway between ordinary sitting and standing, with the thighs slanted downward rather than horizontal. The argument for this posture is that dropping the knees opens up the hip angle and allows the pelvis to rotate forward. This increases the curve of the lumbar spine, bringing it closer to an anatomically normal position and reducing disk pressure. This idea does have some merit. In Chapter 8, you did the Knee–Hips Height experiment, and you experienced that dropping the knees does arch the back.

However, there are problems with the tilted seat pan idea. Remember from Chapter 5 the image of the pelvis as a two legged stool. When you sit down, the two sitbones are what rest on the surface of the chair. That is like sitting on a two-legged stool, and it is an essentially unstable arrangement. Since putting a two-legged stood on a slanted floor won't help it balance, sitting on a slanted seat bottom does not address the fundamental problem of pelvic instability. Not only does it not solve the problem of pelvic instability, but sitting on a slanted surface even interferes with the simple solution of using a towel roll. Since your body's weight does not rest squarely on a slanted seat pan, if you do try to use a towel, your body will have a tendency to slide forward and down off the towel. Sitting in the centered posture on a level or slightly slanted surface will work better for using a computer than trying to sit on a highly slanted seat pan.

LIMITATIONS OF AWARENESS

How has it come to pass that such odd postures as the straight up or reclining styles have been thought of as appropriate? The only answer I can think of is that people examining posture and body use are generally limited by their cultural misunderstandings and their own lack of body awareness.[1]

---

1 An interesting book has recently come out that addresses precisely this issue. The author is a sociologist, a teacher of the Alexander Technique of body awareness training, a practitioner of the martial art of T'ai Chi, and a professor of architecture at the University of California at Berkeley. Her book includes a discussion of the social history and meaning of the chair. She points out that many other cultures prefer what she calls "autonomous sitting," an upright posture that does not use a back rest, and she argues that the body is in fact capable of efficient self-support and does not need a back rest in sitting. *The Chair: Rethinking Culture, Body, and Design*. Galen Cranz. WW Norton & Company, New York, 1998.

European-American culture tends to see the body in piecemeal, top-heavy, and peripheral ways. We normally analyze actions in terms of the body parts that seem to be most obviously involved rather than looking at how the body as a whole does every action. We tend to see power and action as residing primarily in the top part of the body, the arms and shoulders. As an example, think of the image of little boys standing and flexing their biceps to show how strong they are. We also tend to see action as residing in the periphery of the body. We think of the legs and arms as being the active components of the body. We walk, run, squat, and kick with our legs. We lift, push, grasp, pull, and hold with our hands/arms.

Our culture teaches us that effort and hardness are good. If you try hard, you get an "A" for effort. If at first you don't succeed, try harder. Our image of good posture is that it is effortful. You have to try hard and sit up *straight*, with your shoulders pulled back, your back braced, and your gut sucked in. Being strong is good, and strength is equated with tension.

Our culture also teaches us to see the body as separate from and less important than the self. It teaches us to ignore the body in favor of the mind, especially in "intellectual" work, such as computer use and academic research. In this way, the body and mind are split and we take a piecemeal view of the self.

We don't normally see movement in holistic terms. We don't see that every part of the body is involved in every movement. We don't initiate our movements from the core of our bodies. We don't see that real skill and power show themselves in ease and grace, not effort and bracing. We don't see that the mind and body are the very same thing. Because of the way we view the body and the self, it makes sense that people's first thoughts in recommending a good sitting posture for computer work would be either to hoist the body into a braced position or to park the body in a well-supported cradle and then ignore most of it while the mind, hands, and eyes work hard.

However, there is another way to think of and experience the body. *Comfort at Your Computer* is based on the view that all movement originates in and is connected to the core of the body and that the whole body/self is fully involved in every movement. It is based on the view that relaxation, fluidity and balance are the sources of power and effective movement. This is not a philosophical point of view. It is simply the expression of a very different experience of living in one's body. I came to this experience and understanding of my body by being yanked out of our normal cultural mindset/body style.

When I first started using a personal computer, I had been practicing Aikido about twenty years. Aikido is a soft, non-violent Japanese martial art, and the basic assumptions underlying Aikido are very different from those of our European movement heritage. Confronting a radically different way of using the body started me on a long-term process of experimentation that broke me loose from the understanding of the body I had unconsciously absorbed in growing up. (See Appendix C for a bit more about my background and how I came to discover the material included in *Comfort at Your Computer*.)

When I started using my computer, I had to figure out how to get comfortable with it. But in analyzing my posture and movement, I was not starting from the typical European-American view of the body. I was starting from twenty years of experimentation I had done on how my body could move in the most powerful, relaxed and balanced ways. Naturally, I saw the problem of sitting at a computer in a very different light.

• • • • • • •

I would guess that the other reason that ineffective postures have been recommended is that the researchers recommending them probably have not really *felt* what they were recommending. Most ergonomics researchers are academicians or clinicians. They are experts in how to use laboratory instruments or in how to treat physical dysfunctions, and they know a lot about the body from an objective, external point of view. However, I imagine they generally are not experts in the internal, personal skills and artistry of body awareness and movement. Without the personal experience of centered body use as a contrast to the more normal body use, it would be hard to notice or feel the problems in the customarily recommended sitting postures.

I had been practicing Aikido and other body awareness processes for seventeen years when one day I finally had a clear experience of the functioning of the pelvis in postural stability and movement efficiency. Even though I had devoted my life to the area of body awareness training, it took me a long time to get to that experience of pelvic balance. And even in the fields of body awareness and martial arts, I have very very rarely seen the role of the pelvis addressed in anything like the way I address it. It takes a good deal of introspective study of the body and just the right kind of movement experiences to happen upon the particular sitting posture recommended in this book. (Don't worry! You won't need to spend years of effort to discover how to sit comfortably at your computer. You are learning from this book in a matter of hours what it took me years to discover on my own.)

Between cultural and personal limitations, it is no wonder that people whose primary interest has been research or clinical practice rather than body and movement awareness training would not have found the posture I am recommending. Expertise in movement and expertise in laboratory research are separate skills, and it takes the presence of both skills—most likely in a team of movement experts and research experts—for appropriate laboratory research in body use.

Laboratory research on how people can sit most comfortably begins with the culturally limited view of the body that most of us share, and it generally ends there as well. People who aren't highly aware of their bodies will not even think of examining certain options and so will not include them in their research.

Ergonomics studies often examine how people actually sit and then recommend what most people do to try to sit comfortably. The studies don't take account of the fact that people who are not truly aware of their bodies may think that something is comfortable when in fact it causes a great deal of strain. An incorrect way of sitting may simply conform to people's ideas of what ought to be comfortable, or they may be used to it, or it may be the least uncomfortable of many uncomfortable sitting postures they've tried. This process of recommending what people actually do instead of teaching them what they truly ought to do often enshrines people's familiar mistakes as the recommended way to sit.

In the body awareness exercises you experienced in earlier chapters, you felt for yourself the balance and ease that the centered sitting posture creates. By staying true to what you experienced in those exercises, you can evaluate the customary recommendations. You can find a sitting posture that will be powerful, sensitive, comfortable, and safe. That will be a good sitting posture.

KEY POINTS

- The *straight up* style of sitting holds the body with right angles at the knees and hips, the legs close together, and the chest elevated. It is our tense, culturally mandated way of pulling the body up into position. It uses the back muscles to position the pelvis and interferes with free breathing.

- The *reclining style* of sitting leans the body back onto a backrest so that the chair supports much of the weight of the torso, and it uses lumbar support to press the lower back into the proper curves. However, it forces the head to be carried forward, which depresses the chest and interferes with breathing. It results in a longer arm reach to the keyboard, which is more fatiguing. It reduces overall body movement and encourages a disembodied way of sitting.

- The centered sitting posture offers a more comfortable and effective alternative to the commonly recommended sitting styles.

- The straight up and reclining sitting styles probably have been thought of as appropriate because of cultural misunderstandings and lack of body awareness.

12

FIVE-SECOND
MOVEMENT BREAKS DURING WORK

K*eep moving!* The less you move, the worse you will feel and the less you will feel like moving. That downward spiral will leave you feeling as vital and alert as a blob of putty.

This chapter will show you a number of different exercises for moving and stretching through different spirals and circles of movement. You will find that these exercises are different from the spontaneous stretching and fidgeting people often do. Those common movements often fail to relax the most tension-filled body parts and get them moving. The exercises included in this chapter are systematic ways of involving your whole body in gentle, restful movements. You may find that in addition to relaxing you, these exercises will energize you. This positive feeling of relaxed vitality can make long hours of work much more comfortable.

You will be able to do these exercises sitting at your desk. Doing a different movement for about five seconds every ten or fifteen minutes will keep you moving and keep you comfortable. The movements are rather varied, and doing them all in rotation will give every part of your body some recuperation time. Don't feel that you need to do the exercises in the order they are described. And, if variations suggest themselves to you as you do the movements, experiment with whatever new movements arise. If they are satisfying, they can become part of your five-second movement breaks.

It is very important not to sit right for very long. That isn't to say that you should sit wrong, but just that you shouldn't sit motionless for extended periods of time. Even with the best body use in the world, sitting for long periods of time in the same position doing the same limited movements will be stressful.

Taking a few seconds for some simple whole-body movements will make you far more comfortable. The time you spend doing the movements will be more than made up for by reduced fatigue and increased productivity. By taking the small amount of time necessary to prevent discomfort and injury, you will be able to keep working more comfortably and get more done than if you had simply kept working without any movement break. And even if you do "waste" some time on these exercises, preventing injuries and medical bills will make the time expenditure worthwhile in the long run.

Remember—you are your own best investment. If you invest just a bit of time in moving, you will reap great dividends of comfort.

One caution I should suggest is not to substitute rest pauses for good workstation setup and intelligent task design. Don't make the mistake of thinking that resting now and again can make up for bad equipment or tasks that require inappropriate body use. Intense work on intelligently designed tasks with good equipment can still be very strenuous. Movement breaks are designed to help you handle necessary strain. They are not for counteracting the effects of unnecessary strain.

Some computer applications have timed "save" reminders, and there are utilities specifically for reminding you to save your work. If you set the reminder to save every ten minutes, during the few seconds it takes to save your work you can do some movements. If you don't have the convenience of save reminders, you can use a kitchen timer instead.

The next chapter will show you a number of exercises you can do at home. They will not take much time, and doing them on a regular basis will make a real difference in how comfortable you are at work. The chapter after that will show you some movement exercises that you can do in three or four minutes during your break periods at work.

The exercises in this and the next two chapters are simple and gentle. They aren't complicated or strenuous. Nonetheless, if you have any specific injuries or chronic physical problems, be careful about what movements you do. You may need to skip various movements or modify them to make them appropriate for you. The key rule is that *nothing should hurt*. If a movement hurts to do, you are doing it wrong or it is not an appropriate movement for you. If you are in doubt as to whether a movement would be safe for you, check with a physician, physical or occupational therapist, somatic educator, or other professional who is knowledgeable about computers, body awareness, movement, and safety.

• • • • • • •

The movement patterns in this and the next two chapters are different from the other exercises in this book. They are not movement experiments that test various ideas about movement and illustrate basic movement principles. They are opportunities to get your body moving.

In all of the exercises in this and the next two chapters, it is important to savor the feel of the movements as you do them. What do I mean by "savor the feel" of the movements? The key idea is that these movements are not stretches in the way we usually think of stretching. What goes through your mind when you hear the word "stretch"? Most people think of pulling on some tight thing until it tears loose and gets longer. But think about the way a cat stretches. You don't see cats pulling on themselves with tension and effort. They put on such a glorious show of sensuous, delicious, effortless enjoyment of the stretch. Feeling your body in a smooth, sensuous way as you do these movements will lead to a comfortable loosening of your body, just what you need to work comfortably.

These movements are not calisthenics. Don't put any effort into doing them. Many people substitute effort for skill, trying to make up for lack of awareness or understanding by forcing their bodies through movements. If you feel tired after doing the movements, you were working too hard. Do much less and you will get much more.

It is very important to do the movements gently, softly, slowly. They are soft music for your body. They are flowers swaying in the soft summer breeze.

Do the exercises in this chapter sitting on a flat, comfortable chair. Start each exercise in the centered sitting position, sitting forward away from the chair back. You will find that not using a towel roll will allow freer movements in some directions. For some of the exercises, you may want to push your chair away from your desk to give yourself a bit of room to move. Some of the exercises ask you to push on the floor with your feet. If your chair has wheels and it rolls when you push, that will make those exercises awkward. The simple solution is to turn your chair around and brace the backrest against your desk.

There are a few ideas and instructions that apply specifically to the first five exercises, which are derived from the Feldenkrais Method® of movement awareness training. Each of these exercises proceeds through a number of simple steps to build up to a single complex final movement. *When you do a movement at your computer, do only the final movement.* That final movement will take only five seconds, but figuring out the movement the first time will take considerably longer. The best way to learn the five movement patterns will be to go through them very slowly, taking fifteen minutes to half an hour to figure out each one and feel what happens in your body as you do the movements.

Follow each movement instruction as it is written. In many instances, you will stop doing one movement, do a new and separate one, and then add the two movements together. In other instances, you will continue with a movement while adding a new piece to it. When you are supposed to add to a current movement, the instructions will say so. If the instructions don't ask you to continue and add, then you know that you are starting with a new and different movement.

When you are first learning the movements, do them with your eyes closed, so you can focus inward on the sensations of the movement. (When you use the movements as work breaks, you can do them with your eyes open or closed, whichever you like best.) Repeat each movement for a minute or so—s l o w l y—gently—and then stop and rest for half a minute or so. Then repeat the movement again for another minute. Rest again and then go on to the next movement.

As you do the movements, don't just repeat them mechanically, but focus on noticing how they feel. Is the movement smooth and continuous, or is it jerky and hesitant? Can you notice where in the movement and where in your body there is tension and jerkiness, and can you let those areas soften and become smoother? Does the movement feel easier on one side of your body or in one direction? Can you let your body find ways of making the movement equal and even, smooth and easy?

The directions for the first five exercises are somewhat intricate. There are a number of ways to get from the printed directions to the movement patterns. You could read the description of each movement, shut your eyes and do the movement, rest, repeat the movement, and rest again. Then you could open your eyes, read the next movement and continue in that fashion. Or you could tape record the instructions with appropriate timing and rest pauses. You could also ask someone else to read the movement descriptions so that you could keep your eyes closed and not have to shift back and forth from verbal thinking to body consciousness.

Now let's try some movements.

PRACTICE: FORWARD ROLLING MOVEMENTS

1–Nod your head up and down.

2–Make the movement more extensive, looking up at the ceiling and down at the floor. Get your chest and back involved in the movement, raising your chest and arching your back when you look up, dropping your chest and rounding your back when you look down.

3–Roll your pelvis back and forth, forward and back. "Forward" is the direction that arches your back (like a swaybacked horse). "Backward" is the direction that rounds your back into a slump.

4–Combine movements #2 and #3, rolling your pelvis back when you look down, and rolling your pelvis forward when you look up.

5–Continue doing movement #4, inhaling when you look up, and exhaling when you look down. Go slowly, in rhythm with your breathing.

6–Sitting still, with your feet about shoulder-width apart, and your hands resting on your thighs, push on the floor with your feet. As you push, let that movement communicate itself to your pelvis so that it rolls backward and you tuck your tail. When you release the push on the floor, roll your pelvis forward and arch your back a bit.

7–Continuing with movement #6, when you push with your feet and tuck your tail, bring your knees toward each other a bit. Since your feet are staying where they are on the floor, you probably won't bring your knees all the way together. When you release the push and arch your back, spread your knees apart.

8–Continuing with movement #7, when you arch your back, look up, spread your knees, and inhale. And when you look down, tuck your tail, bring your knees together, and exhale. This is the final movement.

PRACTICE: ARM AND PELVIS MOVEMENTS

1—Sitting upright and relaxed, gently extend your arms down at your sides as though you were pointing at the floor. Roll your hands/arms, turning your palms forward and backward.

2—Hold your arms out in front of you at about the height of your solar plexus (the area in your chest where your ribs come together in an upside down V). Keeping your arms at about the same height, open them wide, moving each arm out to the side, as though you were standing with your back to a wall and moving your arms to touch the wall. Then close your arms, crossing them over your chest, as though you were hugging yourself (with your right hand by your left shoulder and your left hand by your right shoulder). This opening and closing movement is fairly horizontal. Gently let your palms face upward as you open your arms and downward as you close your arms.

3—Continue with movement #2, but change it so that the arms describe more of a vertical arc back and forth. Start with your arms across your body in the hugging position, but with your hands down by your lower ribs. As you open your arms, move them in an arc that starts by going up and out and finishes by going back and down. As you move your arms down behind you, turn your palms upward. Then reverse the movement and go back to the hugging position. If your chair has armrests that prevent you from dropping your arms down, either move to a different chair or move your arms out more to the side than down.

4—Continue with movement #3, inhaling as you open your arms, exhaling as you close your arms.

5—Continuing with movement #4, as you open your arms, roll your pelvis forward and tip your head upward. As you close your arms, roll your pelvis backward and tip your head down.

6—Continue with movement #5. As you bring your arms in front of you, push with your feet to help tip your pelvis back. You can pull with your feet just the slightest bit as you open your arms and roll your pelvis forward. This is the final movement.

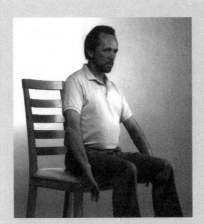

Movement #1.

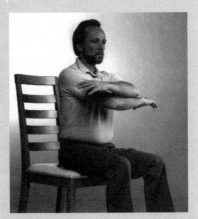

Movement #2.

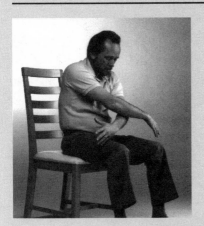

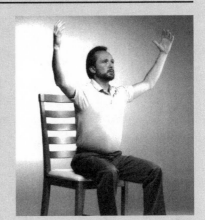

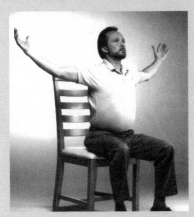

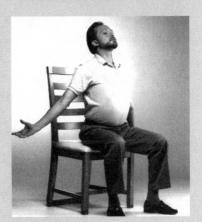

Final movement sequence

PRACTICE: SIDE-TIPPING MOVEMENTS

1–Sit upright, with your feet a bit wider than shoulder-width. Alternate tipping your head to the right and the left. Move your left ear toward your left shoulder, then do the other side. Don't turn your face to the side. Keep facing straight ahead, and just tip your head to the side. Start off with a small movement, just an inch or so to either side.

2–Make the movement larger. Feel how your neck and shoulders become involved in the movement. Feel how the weight shifts on your sitbones.

3–Push with your right foot, and tip your body to the left just a bit. Don't tip so far that you have to exert any effort to stay up. Let your whole body, from your head to your pelvis, tip to the left as though you were a flagpole. When you tip to the left, your weight should go onto your left sitbone. Keep your body straight when you tip, but don't tighten up. Just tip easily.

4–Try pushing with your left foot to tip your body to the right. And then alternate going from side to side. Notice that you shift your weight from sitbone to sitbone as you go back and forth.

5–As you go back and forth, begin to let your head travel farther, so that rather than tipping like a straight pole you begin to bend your body sideways into a curve. Make sure that you lengthen your body to bend to the side. When you move to the right, lengthen the left side of your body up and to the right. Don't just collapse the right side of your body into a bend.

6–Clasp your hands together with your fingers interlaced, and put your hands palms down on top of your head. Continue with movement #5, letting the movement go through your arms as well. This is the final movement, and it is a nice stretch for the whole body. Make sure not to go so far to the side that it is an effort to do the movements.

PRACTICE: SIDE-ARCING MOVEMENTS

1–Sit up, with your knees spread a bit apart. Alternate tipping your head to the right and the left. Move your left ear toward your left shoulder, then do the other side. Don't turn your face to the side. Keep facing straight ahead, and just tip your head to the side. Start off with a small movement, just an inch or so to either side.

2–Raise your right sitbone off the chair by hiking up the bone in the right side of your waist (the iliac crest, the bone that is usually called the "hip") toward your right armpit and making your right side concave. Notice that if you push down with your right foot, it will help mobilize your pelvis for the tipping.

3–Continue with movement #2, and in addition tip your head to the right. Notice that as you hike up your right iliac crest and tip your head to the right, your weight goes onto your left sitbone.

4–Then reverse the movement. Push with your left foot to raise your left sitbone off the chair, and tip your head to the left. Then alternate moving from side to side.

5–When your weight is on your right sitbone and your head and torso are bent toward the left, reach out your left arm sideways as though you were trying to reach toward something on the ground about three feet to the side of your chair. Gently stretch your fingers wide apart. When your left arm is stretched out, let your right arm relax. Do the other side, then alternate sides. This is the final movement, and if you are doing it gently and fluidly, it should provide a nice sensuous stretch.

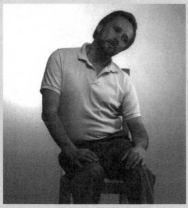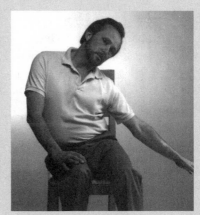

Side-Arcing Movement #4.   *Side-Arcing Movement #5.*

PRACTICE: SPIRAL MOVEMENTS

1—Sitting up, alternate turning your head to the right and the left, as though you are looking at something to either side of you. Start off with a small movement, just a few inches to either side. Let your hands rest comfortably on your thighs, palms down.

2—Keep your head still, and with your eyes closed, look gently from side to side. Make sure that your eyes are soft and gentle as they move back and forth. Normally we turn our heads as well as our eyes to look to the side, but for this movement, use just your eyes. Don't do it as a merely mechanical movement. Feel that you are paying attention to seeing something interesting. Perhaps you are a spectator watching a ball go back and forth in a tennis game. Let your eyes relax and move gently. Don't tense or stiffen to prevent your head from moving. You will probably feel your head move just a bit in sympathy with your eyes.

3—Let your head begin to move in the same direction as your eyes, so you are turning both your head and eyes slowly, right and left, back and forth.

4—Let your torso begin to accompany your head, so that you are turning gently and slowly left and right, turning your chest and shoulders to face to either side. Don't strain to go far. Just do it as an easy movement.

5—Begin moving from your feet. Spread your legs apart so your feet are on the floor a bit more than shoulder-width apart. Push with your left foot to begin the movement of turning your body toward the right. Turn your pelvis to the side as well as your chest and shoulders. As you turn to the right, move your weight onto your right sitbone and let your left sitbone come up in the air a bit. Turn back to the center, but don't do the movement toward the left. Just repeat going toward the right.

6—Turn to the left. Let the movement start at your right foot, spiral up through your pelvis, move into your spine, and end with the turning of your head and eyes. Let each part of your body turn as far as it can comfortably go. Now try turning alternately to the right and left.

7–Now move along a rising and falling diagonal instead of keeping the movement horizontal. As you turn to the left, look up and behind you, as though you wanted to look at something hanging from the ceiling. And as you turn to the right, slide your movement down the diagonal until you are looking at something on the floor behind you to the right. Use your eyes. Actually look. But remember to keep your *eyes closed* and relaxed as you move.

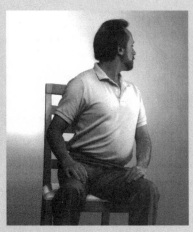

Spiral Movement #6

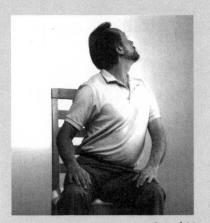 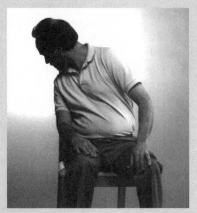

Spiral Movement #7.

8–Now reverse the movement, so that you look up to the right and down to the left. When you look up, inhale, and when you look down, exhale.

9–For the final movement, alternate doing movements #7 and #8, toward the right and left. Do it five or ten times in one direction and then five or ten times in the other direction. Remember to do the movement slowly and gently.

These five movement patterns are ways of moving your whole body. The next few exercise sets will be different from these flowing patterns. They will focus on specific body areas.

PRACTICE: SIMPLE LEG MOVEMENTS

These movements are not a progression. They are separate movements. You can do each one of them for a few seconds occasionally. You don't have to do all of them each time you do any of them. You will, of course, need enough leg room under your desk to move your legs around a bit. All the movements are done sitting up in the centered position.

1—Put your knees about a foot apart. Rapidly, but lightly and gently, flap your knees open and closed for about five seconds. Don't bang your knees together.

2—Come up onto the balls of your feet, as though you were standing on tip toe. And then go down. Do this movement fairly rapidly for about five seconds. Remember to keep the movement light and easy.

3—Raise one foot up, almost straightening your knee. Don't force your knee completely straight. Point your toes and foot forward. Stretch your toes forward, trying to touch the wall. Feel the muscles in your leg tensing. Then, keeping your leg extended, flex your ankle and pull the ball of your foot back. Do this a few times. Then do the other leg. Alternate your legs about four times, not too fast.

4—Raise one foot up and wiggle your toes. Then rotate your ankle, making a circle with your foot. Reverse the direction of the circle. Then do the other foot.

PRACTICE: EYE MOVEMENTS

You can take a few seconds to relax your eyes. These movements are not connected patterns, but isolated movements that you can practice.

1–You might wish to use the Palming Practice (described in Chapter 10) and just rest your eyes.

2–Or you may wish to do some soft, fluid movements of your eyes as described in the Refocusing Your Eyes Practice (in Chapter 10). Close your eyes and move them gently up and down, left and right. Do soft circles one way and then the other. Try some fluid figure eights.

3–The simplest way to relax your eyes is to look off into the distance. Looking across the room or down a hall is helpful, and looking out a window to a distant point is especially good. Shift your focus back and forth a few times. Make sure to soften your eyes as you refocus. Don't strain.

PRACTICE: WRIST STRETCHES

Doing something different with your hands will help relieve the stress of keyboarding. These movements are not connected movements that build to a final pattern, but they do go together as a sequence.

1–WRIST FLEXION: Place your right hand over the back of your left. Hold gently but firmly, grasping the little finger edge of your left hand with your right fingers and the base of your left thumb with your right thumb. Now bend your left wrist to bring the palm of your hand closer to the underside of your wrist. Apply pressure in a smooth, continuous way until you feel a comfortable stretch in your wrist. And then do the other wrist.

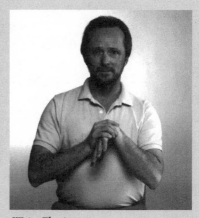

Wrist Flexion.

2–WRIST HYPEREXTENSION:
Hold your left forearm out
in front of you with your
palm facing up and your
elbow bent. Grasp the fingers of your left hand with
your right hand. Do this by
putting your right fingers
across your left fingers and
your right thumb under
your left fingers. Now, pull
your left fingers back while
at the same time straighten-

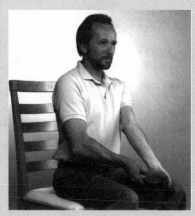

Wrist Hyperextension.

ing your left arm/elbow out in front of you. Then try this on the
other hand.

3–WRIST PRONATION: Hold
your left forearm horizontal
in front of your chest, with
your palm facing away from
you and your elbow bent.
Reach your right hand over
your left. Then grasp the
front of your left hand,
holding the left little finger
edge with your right thumb
and the base of your left
thumb with your right fingers. Now gently but firmly

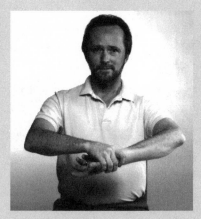

Wrist Pronation.

twist your left hand counterclockwise (so your little finger moves
toward you and your thumb moves away). Do the other hand.

4–WRIST SUPINATION: This is the opposite of Wrist Pronation. Hold your left hand in front of you so your palm faces your face. Your elbow will be bent and low down. Reach around behind your left hand with your right. Hold the base of your left thumb with your right fingers, and put your right thumb on the back of your left hand between your last two knuckles. Now, using your right hand, push with your thumb and pull with your fingers. That will twist your wrist in a clockwise direction. Do the other wrist.

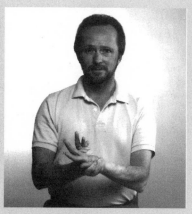

Wrist Supination.

5–Gently grasp each finger and bend it backwards until you experience a comfortable stretch. Do each hand. Then hold your hands down by your sides and shake them, fluidly and gently. Let them flop and wiggle.

Lean back onto the backrest of your chair. Just for a moment, slump, let go. And then sit up and get back to work.

KEY POINTS

- Keep moving. Do a different movement for about five seconds every ten or fifteen minutes. You can use timed save reminders to help you remember to take movement breaks.
- Don't substitute rest breaks or movement breaks for intelligent workstation setup and task design.
- Don't use tension and effort to try to relax. If a movement hurts, you are doing it wrong or it is not an appropriate movement for you.

13

TWENTY-MINUTE
MOVEMENT SESSIONS FOR HOME

The more relaxed and flexible you are, the more easily you will handle the stresses of computer work, the more effective will be the brief movement breaks you take during work, and the more easily you will be able to maintain a comfortable sitting posture. In this chapter, you will learn a series of stretching exercises and two breathing exercises. The exercises will focus on body awareness, relaxation, and flexibility. They will supplement the exercises you do in your five-second computer breaks, and they will provide a foundation for the three-minute movement breaks to be described in the next chapter.

If you do these exercises regularly at home, you will find that they will not be a burden. They will be a pleasure, something you will look forward to and miss if you skip them. Doing them will make you feel relaxed and loose. But if you simply don't have the time to do the exercises at home, don't do them and don't worry about it. The rest of the *Comfort at Your Computer* program will still be effective in helping you attain relaxed and efficient posture.

However, it is important that you go through the exercises in this chapter at least once because what you will learn in this chapter will help you understand how to do the three-minute movement breaks. And I would recommend that you regularly practice the Six Directions breathing exercise for a minute or two even if you don't have time to do the other exercises included in this chapter. It will help you achieve a deep state of alert relaxation.

You may recognize a lot of the stretches in this chapter, but I would like to emphasize some specific ways of doing them that may be new to you. There are a number of important principles that underlie these relaxation and flexibility exercises, but the best way to discuss these principles will be in the context of doing the exercises.

However, before we start the exercises, let me suggest a note of caution. Honor your body's limits. You could be so tight that you can't get even close to a position shown in the photographs. That is fine. Just start where you are and do an abbreviated version of the stretch. Don't feel that you need to stretch as far as the photographs show. If you do just the smallest beginnings of the movements now, you will gradually get more comfortable and do larger movements later. If you need help modifying the stretches to make them more appropriate for you, find a movement professional who can help you with that.

The best surface on which to do the stretching exercises will be a carpet or an exercise mat. You would probably feel uncomfortable doing them on a hard floor, and a soft surface like a bed wouldn't offer enough support.

PRACTICE #1: FORWARD BEND

Take a look at the photograph of the first stretch. The most important thing to keep in mind is that stretching is not stretching! What do I mean by this? Let's try an experiment with the first stretch. Sit on the floor with your right leg out in the position shown. If you're tight and can't bend forward as far as the photograph shows, don't. Sit up straighter. Sit up as straight as you need to in order to straighten out your leg on the floor. You can even lean back if you need to. Now, pull back your toes and the ball of your foot. Press the underside of your right knee into the floor. Notice how tense that makes the back of your leg. Keeping it that way, lean forward, trying to bring your chest toward your knee. This is the wrong way to do a stretch. Don't hurt yourself. We're doing it this way just to understand why it is wrong, so move slowly and carefully. How does it feel? Tense and strained, right?

Most people think of stretching as a process in which a tight muscle is pulled on with force to make it longer, like pulling on a tight leather strap until it gets longer. Some people bounce and tug, some people just exert a steady pull, but most people think of stretching exercises as a process of fighting and overcoming the resistance of the body.

Let's try something very different. Lean forward into the stretch. Move slowly and gently, paying attention to what you feel in your body as you move. Notice exactly when you start to experience a sensation of pulling or tension, and notice where you feel it. Most people will feel the stretch sensation in the muscles on the underside of the thigh, though other areas of the body may be the site of your sensations. The sensation of stretch is the signal that some part of your body has gone as far as it comfortably can.

When you notice this pulling sensation, stop moving forward. Back up slowly and gently, just a little bit, until the sensation of tension disappears. Stay in that place, and focus on relaxing the spot where you had felt the sensation of tension. Let it hang loose. Let it soften. Perhaps imagining/feeling that you are breathing into the spot and letting it warm up will help. After a few seconds you will probably feel the muscles in that spot let go and loosen. When they do, you can move forward a bit, slowly and gently. You will find that you go a bit farther before you feel the sensation of stretch. What you have done is to release the muscle tension that was preventing you from moving farther. Tension equals shortness. When you stop shortening your muscles, they can get longer.

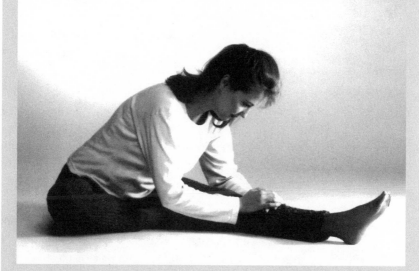

Forward Bend—Lengthened body.

Connective tissue also has its length limits, which are a matter of the organization of the fibers. That organization also has to change to allow greater flexibility. When you release the muscle tension as much as you can, you move to the edge of the connective tissue's limits. At a certain point in your practice of flexibility exercises, after you have felt the release in a given stretch, you will want to exert a small, gentle, steady pull, while continuing to focus on relaxation and release. Doing this will help your connective tissue lengthen as well. You can work with both muscle relaxation and connective tissue change, but you should work only on muscle relaxation until you have mastered that. Later on you can add the gentle pull at the end of the stretch.

This is the first important principle of flexibility training. *Don't force; instead release.*

Do the exercises with the thought that you are learning to release. *Learning* is the key point. Instead of thinking of your muscles as inanimate ropes to be stretched longer, feel your muscles as intelligent and alive. You are teaching them to relax and open up. As you concentrate on experiencing each flexibility exercise in this way, you will become able to utilize a direct releasing/relaxing of any tight spots in your body. You will be able to use each posture as a way of learning to become aware of and take responsibility for how you live in your body.

Sometimes I think I should never use the word "stretch" since it conveys such a tense image. However, it is a convenient word. So I would suggest that when you think of *stretching* exercises, you remember to feel them as freedom exercises.

• • • • • • •

Let's examine more carefully the exact positioning of your body in this first stretch. Notice in the photograph that the back, neck, and head are held long and open instead of hunched-over. Many people do this stretch by pulling the head down toward the knee, but I prefer not to. Pulling your head down and rounding your back compresses your breathing and puts you into a hunched over position. Doing the stretch that way would be teaching you to compress one part of your body while releasing another part. I prefer to confine the action of a stretching posture to one specific part of the body and

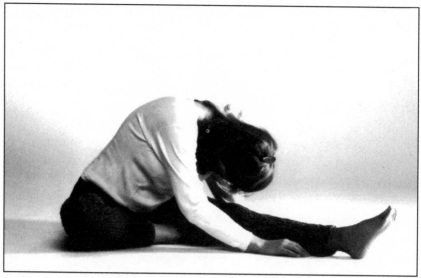

Forward Bend—A compressed, uncomfortable way of doing the stretch.

leave the whole rest of the body as free and open as possible. Each stretching posture focuses on one area of the body, and by doing the group of postures, you will become more familiar with and able to control every part of your body.

Here is the second important principle of flexibility exercises. *Keep the body as a whole in a neutral position and focus each movement on one specific area of the body.*

This first posture focuses on the muscles under the thigh, and there is no reason to drag the rest of the body away from its position of rest and openness. Try to do the flexibility exercises with the same body attitude of length and openness that you practiced in the chapters on sitting and body balance. Doing the postures this way will make them more specific in their action and will help you gain ease and flexibility more rapidly.

• • • • • • •

In any bending movement you do, you can create the movement by shortening one side of your body or by lengthening the other side. When you bend forward in this first flexibility exercise, avoid thinking of shortening your front side. Don't bring your head and chest down. Instead, think of lengthening the back of your body, reaching up, out and over with the back of your body to bend forward. Doing any bend with this lengthening in mind will produce the greatest ease and flexibility. Note that this lengthening is a soft and gentle aiming outward along a smoothly curved line. Don't tense and strain to lengthen.

This is the third principle of effective stretching. *Softly lengthen and open your body into each movement or position.*

As you do the stretch, you are concentrating softly on relaxing. What are you doing with your breathing? Are you paying attention to the sensations of your breath? To relax your body and make most effective use of the stretching postures, your breathing should be soft and full. As described in the Chapter 4, your belly, chest and back should gently swell as you inhale and gently release as you exhale. Your breathing should not be restricted or forced.

The fourth principle is simple. *Your breathing should be full and easy.*

• • • • • • •

These exercises are for you. You are not in competition with anyone, not even yourself. Do not strain or force yourself into any position. Every move should feel comfortable. Go only as far in any posture as feels good to you, and don't strain and pull yourself farther than is absolutely easy and comfortable. Work with what you feel. Discover what each exercise has to teach you.

If you have any physical problems or have had any major injuries, think about whether any specific posture puts strain on a weak area of your body. If you aren't sure whether you should do any or all of these stretches, seek out a professional who can give you advice, perhaps a physical therapist or a body or movement awareness instructor.

The fifth principle is very important. *Don't fight yourself, and don't hurt yourself.*

If you keep these principles in mind as you do all the movements in this chapter, you will find they will be comfortable, helpful, enjoyable and fun.

PRACTICE #2: SIDE BEND

This is a side stretch. You start in much the same position as the Forward Bend, but then you put your back hand on your waist (by the bone ordinarily called your "hip); rotate your torso a bit; and lean up, out, and over to touch your foot. If you can't reach your foot, don't worry. Let your hand rest on your leg wherever it does reach easily.

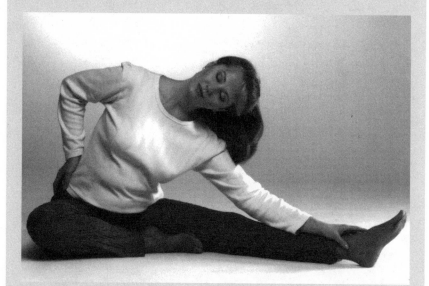

Side Bend.

PRACTICE #3: THIGH STRETCH

This is not a hurdler's stretch. Notice that the foot is tucked in, not turned outward. If you leave your foot turned outward when you lean back, that will twist your knee and could injure it. Tuck your foot in, and lean gently back only as far as is comfortable. Make sure you don't feel any strain in your low back as you do this stretch. Lean your weight onto your rear arm. You can sit up high to reduce the stretch you feel or drop back lower to increase the stretch. (It is especially important not to stretch by kneeling on both knees and leaning back. With both knees tucked, the psoas on each side will be tightened and will pull on your back. This force can actually cause back strain or injury.)

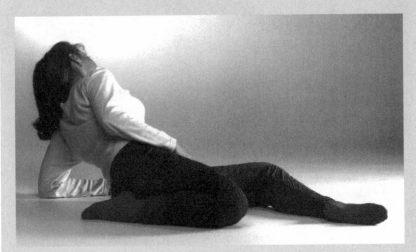

Thigh Stretch.

PRACTICE #4: NECK BEND

People often do a similar stretch in a very different position. They lie on their back and put their legs over their head behind them to touch the floor. That puts considerable weight and compression onto the small vertebrae of the neck, which could cause injury. Sitting up and letting your back round and your head fall gives you a much gentler, safer stretch. If you would like more stretch, interlace your fingers, put your hands up on the back of your head, and allow your elbows to draw your head forward, out, and down. Make sure that you don't tense your shoulders to pull your elbows down. Instead let the relaxed weight of your elbows hang on your hands.

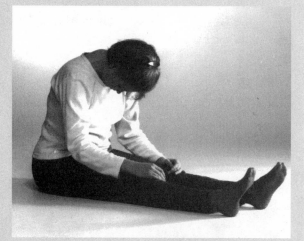

Neck Bend.

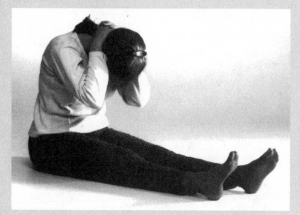

Neck Bend—with more stretch.

PRACTICE #5: BACK ARCH, AND KNEES TO CHEST RESTING POSITION:

Lie on your stomach. Having your feet turned out relaxes your low back and allows an easier stretch. (In Chapter 8, you experienced that opening your legs arches your back a bit, and this is similar.) For a gentle stretch, you can rest on your elbows and let your back/belly hang softly into the floor. For more stretch, you can put your hands on the floor and press up. For less stretch, you can lay your arms flat on the floor, put one fist on top of the other, and rest your forehead on your fists. Make sure you don't feel any discomfort in your back as you do this stretch.

To finish the stretch, lie on your stomach and roll over onto your back. Then bring your knees toward your shoulders, clasp your

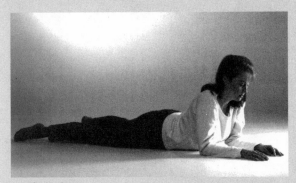

Back Arch.

hands around them, and rest that way for a moment. If you cannot comfortably reach your knees and clasp your hands around them, then just hold each knee with one hand. Resting in this position will relax your lower back further.

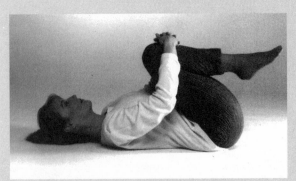

Back Arch—Resting position.

PRACTICE #6:
LEGS SPREAD, CHEST TOWARD THE FLOOR

Spread your legs as wide as is comfortable. Then lean up, out, and over to move forward and bring your chest toward the floor. Remember to lengthen your back and not cave in your body as you do this stretch. If you find it hard to even begin this stretch, another way of doing it may be more comfortable. Spread your legs, put your hands on the floor behind you, and push with your hands. This movement will roll you up over your sitbones, lengthen your back, and stretch your legs.

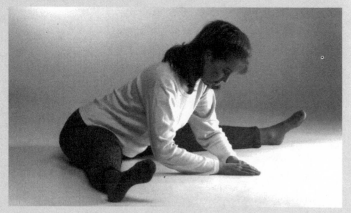

Legs Spread, Chest Toward Floor.

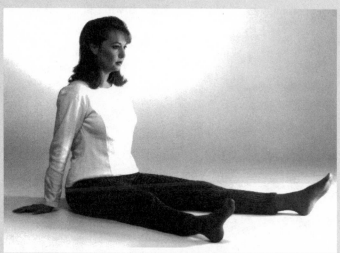

Easier version of Legs Spread, Chest Toward Floor.

PRACTICE #7: SOLES OF FEET TOGETHER, CHEST TOWARD FLOOR

Again, it is important to lengthen, not collapse. Put the soles of your

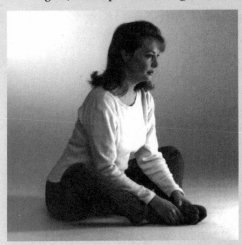

feet together, and bring your feet as close to you as is comfortable. Lean forward, moving your chest toward the floor. Remember to lengthen up and out, and keep your back aligned. If you wish, you can put your elbows on your knees so that your knees will be spread apart as you lean forward.

Soles of Feet Together, Chest Toward Floor.

PRACTICE #8: FOLDED LEGS SPINE TWIST

Sit with your legs folded one in front of the other and your knees on the floor. Reach across to your left knee with your right hand, and pulling on that knee, turn as far as you can go comfortably to the left.

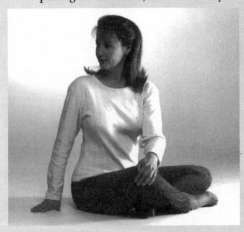

As you turn to stretch, let your back lengthen upward, as though you were a corkscrew spiraling up into the sky. Then do the other side. Of course, if you aren't flexible enough to sit with your legs flat on the floor, don't. Sitting with your ankles crossed and your knees up in the air will be fine.

Folded Legs Spine Twist.

PRACTICE #9: KNEELING

Sit on your heels, with your knees a few inches apart, and with your feet flat on the floor and touching each other. If you are not used to this, don't do it for very long. Just a few seconds may be enough for a start. If you put a pillow between your feet and sit on it as a support for your pelvis, that will take some of the weight off your knees and make the stretch gentler.

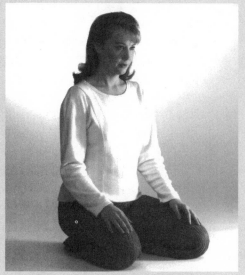

Kneeling.

PRACTICE #10: FOLDED LEGS SITTING, WITH A TOWEL ROLL

If you are flexible enough to achieve this position, you will feel how balanced and stable a posture it is. Sitting this way is very relaxing. It is a good position for doing breathing exercises.

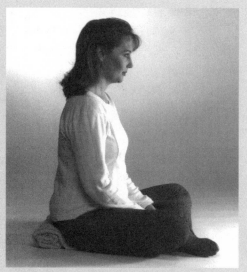

Folded Legs Sitting, With a Towel Roll.

PRACTICE: SIX DIRECTIONS BREATHING

The six directions breathing exercise is a way of practicing the skill of relaxing and balancing your whole body. It is related to the Basic Breathing practice you worked with in Chapter 4. You will use the same sitting posture and the same breathing process, but you will add to that a way of "aiming" your breath as you exhale. The aiming is related to the Pencil Wanting experiment you practiced in Chapter 2. In that exercise you wanted a pencil and felt how that intention to get it actually organized your body for *moving* to go get it.

In the Six Directions Breathing exercise, you will use exhaling in different directions through your body as an image to generate micromovements that will change your overall way of holding your body. You will practice wanting to open your body radiantly outward in a number of directions, and that process of intending to open will actually open your body.

Sit quietly in the centered posture, using a towel for support. You can sit on a chair away from the backrest or sit on the floor with your legs folded. Shut your eyes. As we practiced in Chapter 4, inhale through your nose, drawing the air gently into the core of your body just below your navel. Then exhale through your mouth, relaxing your mouth and throat.

This process of inhaling through your nose and exhaling through your mouth is just for this exercise. Normally you should breathe normally, through your nose. Exhaling through your mouth is a preparation for action, and of course, it is how you breathe when you talk, so breathing in through your nose and out through your mouth in this exercise is a bridge between rest and action.

This exercise will focus on directional imagery as you breathe. When you exhale, imagine that you are gently blowing the air down your spinal column, out your bottom, to a spot six or eight inches (about fifteen centimeters) below you.

Don't just think about this or picture it in your mind, but actually *feel* it in your body, *do* it in your body. Watch out for tipping your head up and rolling your eyes up toward the ceiling as you imagine the path the air takes down through your body. When people look upward, they are usually engaging in an abstract, visual process of imagination rather than an embodied sensation process of imagination. Exhale down for half a dozen or so breaths.

Then change the direction. Imagine/feel that you are exhaling up your spinal column, out the top of your head, to a spot six or eight inches above you. Breathe gently. Don't purse your lips and blow, but just open your mouth, relax your throat, and let the air come out.

After you have done about half-a-dozen breaths, then breathe out of your right side toward a spot about six inches to your right. Next breathe out of your left side. Then breathe to your rear out of your back, and next breathe forward out of the pit of your belly and the front of your body.

For the last breath, breathe in all six directions at once, down and up, left and right, forward and back.

Exhaling a number of times in one direction gives you enough time to really feel how to aim your breath in that direction. However, once you have practiced this whole sequence and felt how it works, there is a more effective way of doing the exercise. Instead of exhaling in one direction for half-a-dozen breaths or so, exhale once in each direction and go through all the breaths in a seven-breath cycle. Always start with the down direction because that is a way of stabilizing the body. Exhale down, up, left, right, backward, and forward. Then exhale in all six directions. And then start the cycle over. You can do this exercise just for a minute or for as much as ten or fifteen minutes—whatever is comfortable and enjoyable for you.

This exercise is a way of practicing keeping an open, even, symmetrical awareness of your whole body. Most people, when they first start working with this exercise, experience that there are areas of their body or directions of their breath that are not clear for them. Any dim spot in the feeling of your body's field of attention is an area of reduced body awareness and reduced vigor. Finding gaps in your field of awareness and breathing life back into them is a way of remembering to live fully in your body. More than that, it is a way of contacting the feeling of living fully in the world. This exercise offers a way of practicing relaxing and balancing your whole body all at once. When you can work at your computer in this way, you will truly be working in comfort. It would be well worth putting a few minutes into doing this exercise every day.

PRACTICE: DEEP REST

A variation on the Six Directions Breathing is very helpful for cram-
ming an hour of rest into ten minutes. You probably would not want
to do this exercise and the Six Directions Breathing exercise one
right after the other since they are very similar. You can do the Deep
Rest exercise by itself any time you need a quick rest.

Lie down on your back. Lie on something firm but padded. A soft
rug on the floor or a firm bed would be fine. Put a pillow under your
head and one under your knees. If your feet tend to flop outward,
your legs might be more comfortable if you pointed your feet
upward and then wrapped a towel around your knees to hold your
legs gently in position. Put your hands on your tummy or on the
floor by your side. Some people find that their arms are most comfortable when they place their hands on their tummies and put a
folded towel under each elbow to raise their arms a bit.

Breathe in through your nose and out through your mouth. Inhale
softly down into your belly. Exhale down into the floor through different areas of your body. Using one breath for each major body segment, exhale down out of your left leg, your right leg, your pelvis,
your back, your right arm, your left arm, and your head. Go through
that sequence a few times, letting your body get heavier and softer
with each exhalation.

Many people find that they get so relaxed from a few minutes of
this that they feel as though they'd slept for hours when they get up.

Here is the last important principle of flexibility and relaxation
work: *Don't hurry and don't worry!*

Don't feel that you are a failure simple because you can't reach
perfect relaxation and flexibility immediately. Progress, not perfection, is the goal. And it may take some time to achieve the progress
you wish in these exercises. You can take your time and learn gradually to be more flexible and relaxed. Also, don't worry if you have
to miss a day or can't put as much time into these exercises as you
would like. Take your time, and improvements will come.

KEY POINTS

- The more relaxed and flexible you are, the more effective your brief movement breaks will be and the more easily you will be able to maintain a comfortable sitting posture.
- As you do your stretching exercises, focus on releasing your body. Keep your body well-aligned and focus each stretch on a particular body area. Lengthen and open your body, and breathe in a full and easy way. Go only as far in a stretch as is right for you.
- Doing the Six Directions Breathing exercise on a regular basis will help you achieve a restful and focused state of relaxed alertness.

14

THREE-MINUTE
MOVEMENT BREAKS FOR THE OFFICE

Some jobs are so narrowly defined that they don't involve anything but sitting at the keyboard all day long, and that can be very stressful. If you are working for long periods of time at your computer, you should have a rest break at least once an hour or so. Depending on how intense the work is, or how boring and draining, you could take a break of ten to fifteen minutes.

Not only does your body need a rest after about an hour of computer work, but so does your mind. It's hard to maintain focused attention for long periods of time. Many people find their concentration slipping after about an hour of work, and their performance declines. If you find yourself getting groggy, distracted, or making more mistakes, a rest break of about ten minutes will help restore your ability to work productively.

Aside from taking a real rest break, getting away from the computer to do some non-computer tasks also offers a change of position and movement. Anything that allows you to do something different for a while offers a chance for reducing computer stress. It would be especially helpful if you have some task that involves walking or moving around.

The time you spend in rest breaks or alternate tasks will vastly increase your comfort and productivity. Taking time for safety and comfort is not wasting time. If you keep working, ignoring your discomfort and fatigue, you will actually get less and less done as you get more and more tired, and you will make more and more mistakes. Taking some time for yourself will let you get more done and get it done better.

On your rest break, you could lean back, shut your eyes, and relax for a few minutes. Or by using the Basic Breathing, Six Directions Breathing or Deep Rest exercises (described in Chapters 4 and 13), you can enter very deep states of focused relaxation very quickly. You could also take time on your rest breaks to get up out of your chair and move around. You could take a walk somewhere or you could do some movement or flexibility exercises.

Here are some simple, basic movements that most people will be able to do quite comfortably. If you have any physical problems, be careful. Think about each of the movements and decide whether you can do it safely. Particularly if you have any back problems, you should be very conservative about choosing what movements to do. Pay attention to your body. If doing some movement is not comfortable, then don't do it. If you have any questions about your ability to do these movements safely, consult a physician or an appropriate movement professional. If for whatever reason you are not able to do these movements, try to find someone knowledgeable about movement who can recommend some other movements that will work for you.

To do these movements, all you need is a clear space next to your desk. The movements will not take much space. They will not be vigorous or get you sweaty. The whole group of movements will take just three minutes to go through, without rushing. Take your time and enjoy them.

These exercises are meant to relax and comfort your body. Don't do the movements vigorously or quickly. They are not calisthenics. Move slowly and softly.

If you are wearing high heels, you will have to take them off to do the exercises safely, but I imagine it will be a relief to take them off for a few minutes. If you are wearing a tight tie and jacket, you will probably want to loosen your tie and take off your jacket.

It is very important to open your body as you do these exercises. You can bend any joint by imagining you are shortening one side or by imagining you are lengthening the other side. If, for example, you bend forward by shortening and collapsing your chest and belly, you will increase the discomfort in your body. If instead you bend forward by lengthening and releasing your whole back, you will open your breathing and relax your muscles.

One last thought about doing these exercises. If you work at home or have an office to yourself, you can simply do the exercises and not be concerned about anyone else's opinions. If you do the exercises in a workspace or lounge that you share with others, you may get some odd looks. Some people just don't want to put out the effort it takes to feel good and would rather spend their time complaining about feeling bad. The couch potatoes in the group may not want to see someone else taking sensible care of themselves. Seeing someone else doing relaxation/movement exercises may make them feel guilty, and they may try to deal with this by making you feel bad about doing the exercises. Just smile and breathe. You will be using your computer comfortably long after they have had to quit using theirs in pain. Perhaps if you keep on enjoying your awareness exercises, they may be moved to think about moving themselves.

● ● ● ● ● ● ●

Honor your body's limits. Don't feel that you need to go as far or do as much as the photographs show. If you do a small movement now, you will gradually get more comfortable and do larger movements later.

PRACTICE: SQUATTING

As you squat down, put your hands down on the floor for balance and stability. If you wish to make the movement easier, hold onto a desk or a chair (a stable one that won't tip) and go only part way down. Try different foot positions to find the most comfortable one. Make sure to keep your knees comfortably apart.

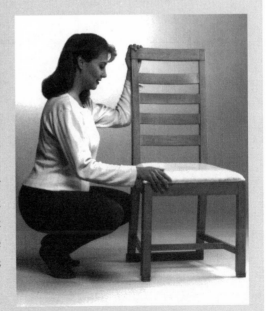

Squatting—holding the chair for support.

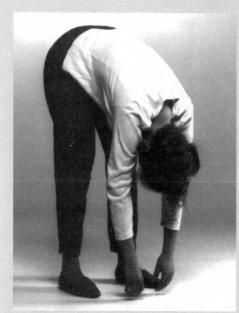

PRACTICE: HANGING

From a standing position, gently let your head fall forward and down, and follow that movement with your back, vertebra by vertebra, until you are hanging forward. Don't get up by just lifting your back. Bend your knees and assume a bit of a squat position, and then rise up from there.

Hanging.

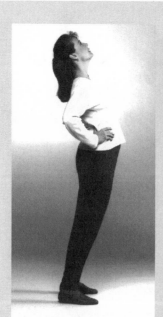

PRACTICE: ARCHING BACK

Standing up, put your hands on your waist and move your belly forward until your back has assumed a gentle arch. Make sure to lengthen your front to assume the arching position. This exercise can be done by moving your shoulders back, but that movement puts more pressure on the back and may be too much for some people.

Arching Back.

PRACTICE: SIDE STRETCH

To stretch to your right, put your right hand on your waist and move your pelvis toward the left. Let your head bend to the right. If you want more stretch, you could reach up and out to the right with your left hand. Then do the other side.

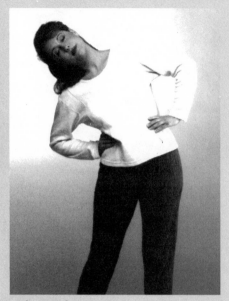

Side Stretch.

PRACTICE: BACK OF THE LEG STRETCH

Lean against a wall or desk with both hands. Keep one leg back, and make sure that the foot of that leg points straight forward, not out to the side. Then lean forward into the wall and lengthen your back heel into the floor. You will feel a stretch along the back of your back leg.

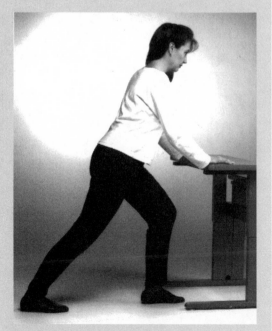

Back of the Leg Stretch.

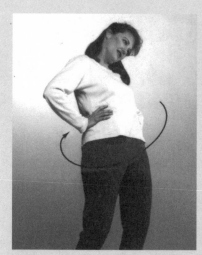

Pelvis circles.

PRACTICE: PELVIS CIRCLES

Stand with your feet fairly close together and your hands on your waist. Imagine that you have a sponge tied to each side of your pelvis (on what would ordinarily be called your "hips"), and you are standing inside a big wooden barrel. If you move your pelvis around in a circle, you will be able to sponge out the inside of the barrel. Make sure to alternate the direction of the circles.

PRACTICE: LEG SWINGS

Hold onto a desk or put your hands against a wall. Now swing one leg gently forward and backward. Make sure that the movement is not too vigorous and that you don't swing your leg so far back that it overarches and compresses your lower back.

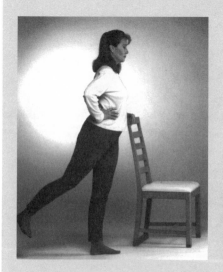
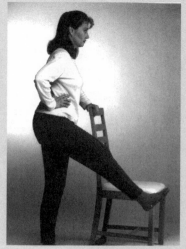

Leg Swings—Holding the chair for balance.

PRACTICE: ARM CIRCLES

Swing your arms back and forth, out to the sides, and then across your chest.

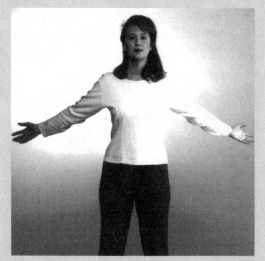
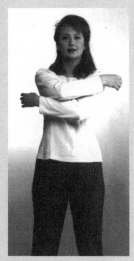

Arm Circles #1: Back and forth.

Next swing them in circles across your front, going first in one direction, then reversing the direction. Move at a gentle, comfortable speed. Let the circles described by your wrists cross in front. If you keep your arms far enough apart that the circles don't cross, that will be less comfortable.

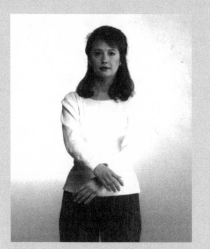
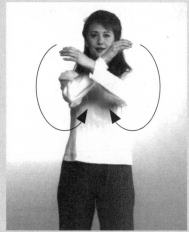

Arm Circles #2: Large Circles.

PRACTICE: HEAD MOVEMENTS

Standing up, nod your head up and down. Make sure that you don't collapse and compress the back of your neck when your chin goes up. Turn your head right and left. And tip your head to your right shoulder and then to your left shoulder. Make sure to lengthen your neck gently as you do these movements.

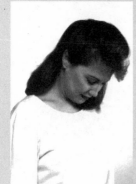
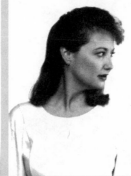
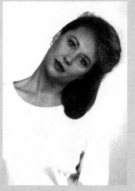

Nodding.   *Turning.*   *Tipping.*

KEY POINTS

- Take a break from your work every hour or so, for five, ten, or fifteen minutes, depending on how strenuous your work is.
- For a change of position and movement, get away from your computer to do some non-computer tasks.
- Take some time for whole-body, large movements. Do only as much in the movements as is right for you. Lengthen and release your body in each movement.

PART II

YOUR WORK ENVIRONMENT

15

MAKING YOUR DESKTOP
WORKSTATION COMFORTABLE

Now it's time to apply the body awareness you have gained to the challenge of setting up your workstation. We will start by analyzing the desktop workstation, but the material in this chapter will provide a foundation for the discussion of both laptops and standing workstations.

How should you set up or adjust your workstation? There is a very simple answer. Your work environment should be adjusted to you. It should support you in your position of comfort. You should never have to adjust to your work environment and distort your posture or movement.

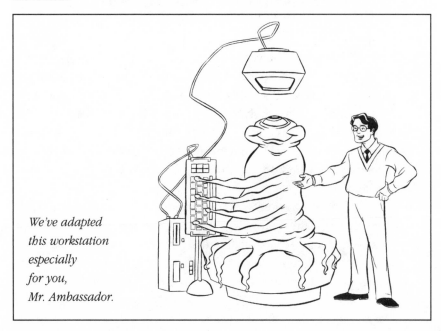

*We've adapted
this workstation
especially
for you,
Mr. Ambassador.*

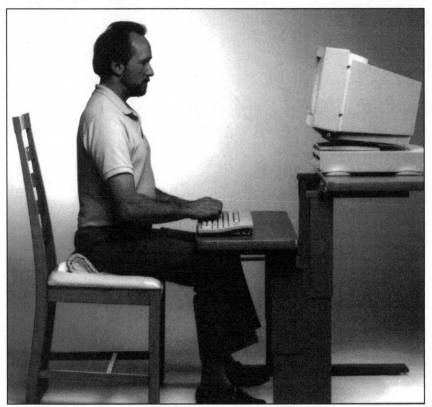

Comfortable, centered body use at a desktop workstation.

That is a simple answer, but far from satisfactory. You have completed your tour of your body, and you can feel what your body needs for comfort. But where exactly should you place your computer, your desk, your chair, and so on? What is the best chair for you? Knowing your body is just the beginning. Now it's time to apply that knowledge to your equipment. The rest of the book will focus specifically on how to set up and use your computer and related equipment.

All of the suggestions in this chapter and the next two will stem directly from the body awareness information presented in the first section of the book. Rather than writing the suggestions in the form of experiments, for simplicity I will simply state what I have experienced to be the best ways to work with computers. Now that you have gotten used to the process of body/movement experimentation, you can always test the suggestions for yourself and see what feels best by comparing them to their opposites or to various alternatives.

Remember that our focus in this book is primarily on body awareness and posture. There is a lot of material available about elements such as office layout and air quality, and all of that is important in creating a comfortable and healthful work environment. However, what has not previously been available is a careful consideration of the body awareness elements of workstation design, and that will continue to be the focus here.

There are two ways to approach body awareness and workstation adjustment. Now that you know how your body works, you may be able to get comfortable with the equipment you have, or you can go out and buy new and better equipment. You may do either or both, depending on time and financial constraints.

If you do not run your own business, decisions about your workstation may not be altogether up to you. You may have to contend with rules in your workplace about office decor and how you are allowed to set up your workstation. You will almost certainly have to deal with people who do not have the understanding of workstation design you have gained from this book and who in any case will limit the amount of money you can spend on workstation improvements. Make sure to point out that the time and money the company puts into comfort and safety will be more than paid for with increased productivity and reduced medical bills.

However, remember the key idea of this whole book—body awareness. Ergonomically correct furniture is important. Yet if you don't remember to use your body efficiently and gracefully, then even the best chair in the world won't "fix" your strain. And if you do use your body well, you may not even need costly new equipment.

GENERAL POINTS

There are some general points to consider about the comfortable use of your computer. First, don't get angry at your computer. Sometimes it seems that your computer is out to get you. Other times, when you are a bit more rational, you know your computer is just a hunk of silicon and metal, but it can be a terribly frustrating machine. Remember to use the relaxation and body awareness exercises you have learned to prevent the physical strain that frustration will cause.

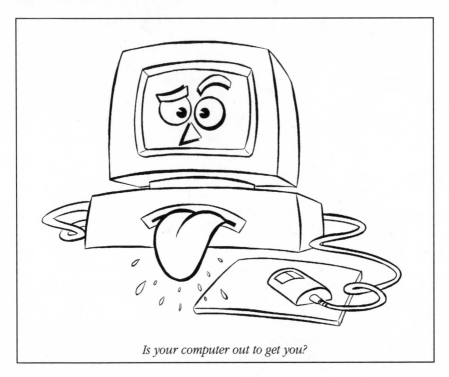

Is your computer out to get you?

One suggestion for reducing frustration is to use your hardware and software manuals. I know that reading manuals takes time and that it seems more masterful to plunge straight into the jungle and survive. Still, by reading manuals you can learn the easiest and most efficient ways to use your computer and software, and that will help you avoid frustration and stress. You may also find it helpful to subscribe to a computer magazine and to join a computer users' group. The more you learn and the more resources you have, the easier your computer work will become.

Think about the layout of your workstation. Pay attention to the aesthetics and neatness of your workspace. A well-organized and uncluttered space will feel more comfortable. Organization has its practical benefits as well. The items that are most important and that you use most frequently should be in places that are easy to reach so you won't be tempted to lean over in awkward positions to get them.

Ideally, most of your workstation equipment should be adjustable. It will be important to read the directions and know how to adjust your equipment. The controls on equipment should be accessible from your normal work position. If you have to get out of your normal work position to adjust something, you won't be able to tell how the adjustment affects you until you get back to work. That up and down process of adjustment is inefficient at best. The controls should be easy to understand and use.

The most important point to keep in mind is that if you try for perfection, you are guaranteed to fail. It is true that the standard I hold up for good sitting is perfect balance and comfort. However, that is just an ideal, a way to provide a direction for our work. In real life, you will have many tasks and many competing requirements for positioning and moving. Do the best you can, but don't feel defeated by the fact that it is never possible to set up your workstation *perfectly*.

CHAIR

Your chair is the most fundamental element of your workstation setup. It directly shapes your sitting posture. It either supports you well or makes your work life torture.

It is possible to find a comfortable chair, one that allows you to be you. The chair should be neutral. It shouldn't force you into odd positions but should allow you to use your body in a centered way.

I once conducted a demonstration of body awareness training for my computer users group, and the person who volunteered for the demonstration of proper sitting posture happened to be wearing a TENS unit (an electrical gadget for interfering with nerve transmission of extreme chronic pain). Once I helped her into her position of comfortable balance, she exclaimed with great surprise that the simple plastic cafeteria chair she was sitting on felt better than the $600 ergonomic chair she had tried out just the day before. The chair did not feel better. She felt better on the chair. That was the secret.

In the earlier chapters on body awareness and posture, you experienced what comfortable, relaxed, alert sitting is. There are two primary sources of discomfort in sitting: pressure and muscle work. If body weight rests on a surface, then there will be pressure on the part of the body part touching the surface. That pressure can irritate nerves or other body tissues and cut off free blood flow. If you hold your body in a given position for a long time, that will fatigue and irritate your muscles. People often fidget when they get uncomfortable in an unconscious attempt to change the amount and location of the pressure they experience and the work they do. A good chair will minimize both pressure and work, making it possible to work comfortably for greater periods of time.

What should you look for when picking out a chair? I recently had an interesting conversation with a woman responsible for choosing new chairs for a large organization. Many of her employees were complaining about the chairs they had. Some of her employees had been to the firm that did their accounting and had found the chairs used there very comfortable. They had asked her to purchase the same chairs for her organization, so she phoned the accounting firm to find out what they had. What they had was a problem! The employees who used the chairs found them very uncomfortable and were demanding new chairs. The moral of the story is that what feels good to sit in for five minutes may be very uncomfortable after five hours. You have to know your body and have some idea of what to look for to pick out a chair that will be comfortable and safe in the long run.

CHAIR HEIGHT: The first thing to look at is chair height, and the correct height is determined by your body dimensions (see Chapter 8). The distance from the floor to the top surface of the seat pan should be equal to the distance from the sole of your foot to the underside of your thigh. Of course, if you wear shoes while you type, the thickness

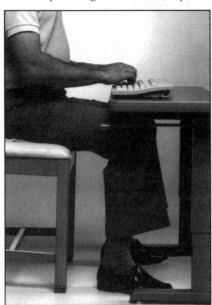

of the sole of your shoe must be added to the length of your leg. If the height of the seat pan is greater than the length of your lower leg, your feet will dangle instead of being firmly planted on the floor. That will reduce postural stability. It will also put pressure on the undersides of your thighs, pressing on nerves and cutting off free blood circulation, which will lead to discomfort and ultimately to physical damage. If the height is not great enough, your knees will be raised too high relative to your pelvis. That will roll your pelvis back and destroy the firm foundation for your posture.

Chair height is determined by the length of the lower leg.

It is simplest, of course, to use adjustable chairs. However, if your chair height isn't adjustable, you must find a way to create adjustments. If your chair is too low, you must raise the seat pan. On some chairs, depending on how the seat pan is attached, it would be possible to put blocks under the seat pan to raise it. Or you can raise the chair by placing blocks under the chair legs—but make sure the chair is stable and won't fall off the blocks. The simplest solution is to use a firm, neutral-shaped seat cushion. Having a supply of seat cushions of different thicknesses would be especially helpful in schools, where students of different ages and sizes all have to sit at the same computers.

If the chair is too low, you could also put plywood sheets under the chair to raise it up. Use as many thicknesses of plywood as you need to gain the required height. However, if your chair is on wheels, putting it on a plywood sheet creates a situation in which you may roll back off the sheet. That could tip your chair and lead to a fall. If your chair is on wheels, nail a strip of wood around the edge of the plywood to keep your chair on the platform.

If your chair is too high, then you must lower the seat pan. If it is the kind of chair that has four legs, you may be able to cut a bit off each leg to lower the chair. The simplest solution is to use a foot rest to bring the floor up to your feet. It is easy to make footrests with plywood, or you can buy them. Again, for schools it would be helpful to have a supply of footrests of different heights.

HIGH HEELS: The discussion of chair height presumes that your feet will rest flat on the floor, which is the position of comfortable support (see Chapter 8). If you wear high heels, that will raise your heels and effectively increase the length of your lower leg plus shoe. And it will do that while dropping your toes. I understand that for many business situations it is simply necessary to fit the mold and wear high heels. Nonetheless, there is no way to be as comfortable as possible at your computer while subjecting your feet to high heels. Some people use a foot support and let the heels dangle off the edge, but that raises the legs and requires that the chair and desk be a different height as well. Given a choice, you should avoid high heels, and if you don't have a choice, wear the lowest heels possible or remove them when working at your computer.

SEAT PAN ANGLE: What angle should the seat pan be set at? Should it tilt back, be level, or tilt forward? There is a common idea that the seat pan should be tilted back so that the body's weight falls onto, and is supported by, the backrest. Leaning back tends to force your pelvis to slide forward, thereby rounding and creating compression in your back. The lumbar supports on rear-tilted backrests are supposed to deal with this problem by pushing the spinal column back into its normal curves, but that applies only to the low back. Leaning back also distorts the use of your upper spinal column. It thrusts your head forward (see Chapters 5 and 11), which creates strain on your neck and interferes with your breathing and with free movement of your shoulders and arms.

There are two chair styles in which the seat pan slants forward. In the first style, an essentially ordinary chair has a pronounced forward tilt of the seat pan and places you in a half-standing posture. Some people put a foam wedge on an ordinary chair to arrive at the same tilt. How does that affect your sitting posture? Remember the image

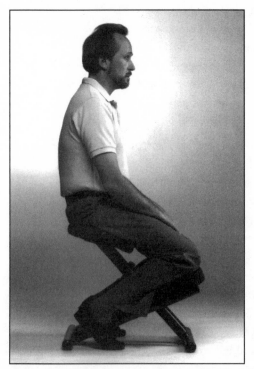

of the pelvis as a two-legged stool (discussed in Chapter 11). Putting a two-legged stool on a tilted surface won't help its balance, and tilting a seat pan forward won't result in better pelvic balance. When people sit in such a chair, they tend to slump, just as they would on an ordinary chair. If the tilt is very great, there will also be a tendency for you to slide forward off the chair. That will have to be prevented either by using rough fabric to provide friction or by bracing your feet against the floor, but bracing with your legs will create strain and discomfort.

A kneeling chair does not create good sitting posture.

The other chair style that has a forward tilting seat pan places you in a position which is midway between kneeling on your knees and sitting. The seat pan is tilted forward quite a bit and your knees are positioned against padded braces to prevent you from sliding forward off the chair. In order to write this paragraph with the greatest possible authenticity, I moved onto such a chair. I am sitting on one of these chairs as I type this, and it is quite uncomfortable. The tilted seat pan doesn't help me avoid slumping. Even with a towel under my tailbone, I cannot get my body into the upright and balanced position we have worked on. The tilted seat pan and the bracing of my knees prevent easy adjustment of my body. My feet are tucked underneath me and there is uncomfortable pressure against my toes.

Safety and comfort in computer sitting demand movement, but this style of chair wedges you into position and prevents free and easy movement. Not only that, but it puts direct pressure on your knees and indirect pressure on your hips, which leads to discomfort. Also, many such chairs are not adjustable. They put you into a fixed and somewhat contorted position, and it would even be hard to add height to the seat pan by putting down pillows to sit on. I'm going to get off this chair now. It simply isn't comfortable.

The best angle for the seat pan is a very minimal tilt forward. Your knees should be slightly lower than your hips in order to encourage proper pelvic rotation. And of course you should use a towel roll to support your pelvis in proper rotation. If your chair is level or slants back just a bit, you may be able adjust it by putting a piece of plywood under the rear legs of the chair to raise them up a bit.

PADDING: The seat pan should be padded to cushion your sitbones. If you sit for a long time on a hard surface, the flesh under your sitbones will get sore. But padding that is too soft allows your body to sink into it. That won't offer enough postural support. It will also inhibit movement, which will make it hard to stay comfortable. A chair that may seem cushy and comfortable for five minutes of sitting can wind up being torture over long hours of work.

The padding should be firm enough for good support and soft enough to absorb weight, but not so soft that it bottoms out and puts your weight onto the hard surface of the chair. The covering for the padding should be of fabric that breathes so you don't get hot, sweaty, and sticky.

TOWEL ROLL: While we are on the topic of padding, let's consider the towel. I recommend a rolled up towel primarily because bath towels offer better support than anything else I have found. They are firm but soft and conform well to the shape of your bottom. They breathe, and they are very easy to shape. I haven't found any foam rubber that is as easy to use as a towel. However, make sure that the towel you use really is comfortable, both in firmness and shape. If the towel is too thick, unroll it a bit and sit on what's left. If the towel is too tight and firm, it might actually make your tailbone sore. And if you are sitting on a slick surface, to prevent the towel from rolling backward out from under your tailbone, unroll it a bit and put the unrolled portion under your sitbones.

SEAT PAN SHAPE: The shape of the seat pan is also important. Many seat pans are contoured, but I find that prevents free and easy movement. In the proper pelvic alignment, with a towel for support, the contouring doesn't offer any advantages. A flat seat pan allows people of every different sizes and shapes to find their own comfortable sitting postures. If your chair is bucket-shaped or contoured, you can remedy that by filling in the low spots with towels.

A rounded soft edge on the front of the seat is very important. A sharp edge would create a lot of pressure on the underside of the thigh, cutting off blood flow and irritating skin, muscles, and nerves. A rounded, soft edge prevents this.

For most people, when they sit upright without leaning back on the backrest of the chair, the length of the seat pan is not an issue. Some very tall people might find that a longer seat pan gives their thighs more support. However, it is important to remember that a seat is not just good or bad. It is good or bad *for something*. If you are brainstorming on the telephone, there is no compelling reason to sit upright in the posture that would be most effective for typing. You can lean back, and in that situation, the length of the seat pan would be important. It should be short enough that you can lean back on the backrest and simultaneously touch the floor comfortably with your feet.

BACKREST: I do actually recommend that your chair have a backrest. You should not spend too much time sitting motionless even in the correct posture. You should be able to lean back occasionally for a change of position. When you want to lean back and contemplate your navel, the universe, blowing up your computer, or all of the above, you can use the chair's backrest. You might even want to lean back and type for a few minutes just for a change—though I find that so uncomfortable that I almost never do it. If you do lean back against the backrest, don't collapse your body. Keep your back lengthened and open.

The backrest on your chair should be padded. Lumbar support is helpful when you use a backrest, and it is best if the position and thickness of the lumbar pad is adjustable. (The lumbar curve is the small of your back, the inwardly curved area just above your waist.) Of course, you could place a pillow or folded towel behind yourself to adjust the location of the support offered for your back.

WHEELS: Chairs with wheels allow you to move back and forth between different task areas at your workstation. However, if your chair rolls too loosely on its wheels, that could be problematic, especially on slick hard floors. I encountered this situation with two different computer users in one week. Both had offices that were in nice old buildings. The buildings had settled a bit over the years, and the hardwood floors were noticeably tilted. Both computer users had to press into the floor with their feet and tense their whole bodies simply to prevent their chairs from rolling away from their desks. And they felt awful by the end of the day. If your feet cannot rest in a relaxed, firm and comfortable manner on the ground, your legs and low back will get very tense.

Some chairs roll so easily that even on flat floors the pressure of your legs against the ground will tend to roll your chair away from your desk. With such chairs, rather than letting your feet settle into the floor, you have to lift your legs a bit to reduce their pressure on the ground. If your chair rolls too easily, that can be solved by using a chair that doesn't have any wheels, by locking or tightening your chair's wheels if that is possible, or by putting a carpet underneath to keep your chair from rolling.

SECRETARY'S CHAIR: The most uncomfortable possible chair is the old-style "secretary's" chair. It may roll loosely on its wheels so your feet cannot rest firmly on the ground. It often is not adjustable in any way. The backrest may be positioned so high that it doesn't offer good lumbar support. The backrest may even fall back when you lean on it, and the seat pan may tip back as well. Such a chair provides no support at all for your back and especially for your pelvis. It encourages a sitting position in which your pelvis rolls back and your chest caves in. It encourages strain and fatigue. If you have such a chair and you find there is no way to adjust and stabilize it so it gives you firm support, then dispose of it. Perhaps you could turn it into a lamp or a paperweight or something of the sort.

ARMRESTS: Sitting in the centered posture, your elbows will hang comfortably by your sides, and your keyboard should be just a bit farther from your body than the length of your forearms (see Chapter 7). If your chair does have armrests, they should not hit your desk and prevent you from pulling your chair as close to your computer table as you need to. For sitting and typing, you will probably not need any arm rests at all. Some short-torsoed people will find their elbows hitting the armrests when they sit in the centered position, and they will need chairs without armrests.

If you recline in your chair or sit too far away from your desk, then you will have to reach out toward your keyboard, and you may well feel a need to use armrests to keep the weight of your arms from dragging your shoulders and chest down into a slump. You may be sitting too far away because your chair's armrests are too high and prevent your chair from sliding under your table or desk. In other words, arm rests that don't fit under your desk make you sit so far away that you may need the armrests to hold up your arms. It would be better just to make sure your armrests fit under your desk.

If you do use armrests for typing or for non-computer activities, the arm rests should be adjustable so they can be placed at the height at which your forearms naturally rest. That height will, of course, depend on what sitting posture you are using and what activity you are engaged in. If you do rest your arms on armrests, make sure that the armrests are soft enough that you don't irritate your arms by constant pressure on the same areas over long periods of time.

SADDLE SITTING: There is one last sitting option that may seem odd but which I use a lot and find quite comfortable. I often sit on a stool that has a rolled up blanket on it. It is very similar to riding horseback and sitting on a saddle. The blanket roll points forward, just as the spinal column on a horse does. Rather than sitting on a flat surface as with a customary chair, this has you sitting on a somewhat rounded surface. Your legs are spread apart. The blanket is a bit higher than a seat pan would usually be, so your knees are a bit lower than usual, which encourages a slight arching of your back. This sitting posture allows your legs and pelvis to find a natural, relaxed stability, which enables them to support your torso in a comfortable manner. It also encourages a very comfortable opening and relaxation of your breathing.

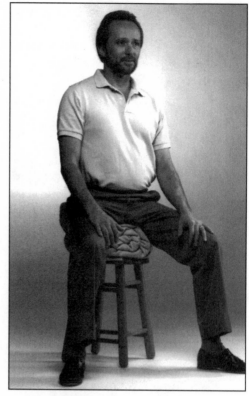

Saddle sitting can be quite comfortable.

DESK

After your chair, your desk is the next most important piece of workstation equipment. Your chair supports you, and your desk supports your work.

DETERMINING HEIGHT: Writing, reading, or keyboarding require somewhat different desk heights and arrangements. However, the height of your desk surface is determined primarily by your seated height. Once you have adjusted your chair to your body requirements, you will know what position your body will be in as you work, and you can determine how to place your desk to support that body position.

The desk surface has to be at the height that will allow your hands and arms to maintain their optimal positions. For keyboarding, you will be sitting in the centered position, with your elbows hanging by

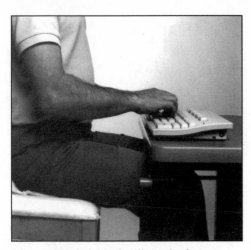

The correct desk height allows the forearms to be horizontal and the wrists to be straight.

your sides and your forearms out in front of you horizontally. The desk should be the right height to place the keyboard right under your fingers.

If your desk is too low, you will not be able to position the keyboard where you need it for comfortable typing. You will have to lean over to type. If your desk is too high, you will have to hold your arms too high. In either case, you will feel strain and fatigue in your back, neck, and shoulders.

ADJUSTING HEIGHT: If your desk does not support your work in the position needed by your body, then you will have to raise or lower the desk to meet your requirements. Ideally, your desk should have a mechanism to allow you to adjust its height. If you do not have such a high tech desk, you will have resort to some low tech adjustments.

To raise your desk, put wooden blocks or something of the sort under the legs. Of course, you must make sure that the blocks will offer stable and safe support. You can purchase desk risers instead of using wooden blocks. (See the Resources listing at the end of this chapter.)

To lower your desk, you could cut a bit off the legs, but the chances are that will not be possible. You may not be allowed to perform major surgery on the office equipment, or the desk may be built so that cutting it down is difficult or impossible. Instead, you can raise yourself up. The simplest solution would be to put enough layers of plywood under your chair to raise you as high as you need to go. The plywood will have to be large enough that you have room to put your feet on it and room to move your chair as you sit down at your desk and stand up from it. If your chair is on wheels, be careful not to roll back and fall off the plywood. It would be safest to nail a strip of wood around the edge of the plywood to keep your chair on the platform.

In schools, computers are often placed on adult-sized tables or desks, and typically the children will need to sit higher up. Since many different children of different ages and sizes have to use the computers, the simplest solution will be to have a supply of various-sized cushions and footrests.

WRITING: Setting up a desk for computer use involves different height requirements than setting up a desk for writing on paper documents by hand. In writing, your arm will be positioned much as it would be for keyboard work, but the thickness of the keyboard will be absent, and so the desk will have to be that much higher for comfortable arm use. Writing on a desk that is adjusted for keyboard work will force you to lean down just a bit, and that will strain your arm and neck.

You might notice as you write where you position your paper. Many people center it in front of themselves on an extreme angle and then twist their bodies around. If you were right handed, that would mean putting the paper in front of you, positioned so that the left top corner is farther to the left than the left bottom corner. Then you would twist to your left to get your arm into position on the paper. Try putting your paper off to your right side, facing almost squarely ahead, with just a bit of slant to the left. In that position, your writing arm and your whole body will be much more comfortable. (For more information about body use and writing, and for a photograph of the recommended writing position, see the section later in this chapter on graphics tablets.)

If you do both extensive writing and extensive computer work separately from each other, ideally you would have different work surfaces for each activity. You could have a desk with two different work surfaces, or you could have a writing table placed right next to your computer desk. If you have just one work surface, then you will have to adjust either the keyboard placement or the writing surface. If you have your desk designed to fit your keyboarding requirements, you can get a slab of smooth wood the same thickness as your keyboard on which to write. Of course, you will have to make sure that you don't lean your forearm on the edge of the wood. If you do, the constant pressure will wind up being quite uncomfortable and possibly injurious.

If you choose to have your desk fit your writing height require-ments, there are retractable shelves that can be affixed to your desk to hold your keyboard in front of and lower than your desk surface height. Of course, putting your keyboard on a shelf in front of your desk necessitates moving your chair and affects the positioning of your monitor (which will be discussed shortly).

DESK SPACE: In addition to desk height, the space on your desk is important. The primary consideration is that your monitor should be about an arm's length from you. Your desk has to be large enough to accommodate the monitor and still get it far enough away from you for proper viewing. You may also have your computer on your desk, though some computers can be placed on the floor or else-where out of the way.

Your desk has to be large enough to hold whatever other tools you use. That may include a telephone, calculator, printer, container for floppy disks, postage scale, bin of paper, etc. You will also need space for your paper documents, both those that you read and those you write on. You may also need space to keep manuals open. (We will discuss document placement later in this chapter.)

Everything on your desk should be arranged so that you can reach what you need without stretching or twisting uncomfortably. In order to increase your available desk space, you may want a desk with a table right next to it. And you may want a chair that swivels and rolls, which would allow you to turn from your desk to your table, pro-viding of course that it isn't so mobile that it does not allow for pos-tural stability.

LEG SPACE: Another element to consider is the amount of room avail-able for leg movement. Does your desk have enough free space underneath that you can move your legs around? This is especially important to consider if there are drawers under the desk surface, if you are using a keyboard shelf, or if you have very long legs. If your feet are confined, you will experience tension in your legs, and that tension will affect every part of your body and make you tense all over. Even though the most stable posture is one in which your feet are flat on the floor under you, you should still move your legs to other positions for a moment as you type or while you rest, just for the sake of changing your posture and keeping your legs from being stationary too long.

While we are talking about what goes on under your desk, think for a moment about your feet. It is best to wear comfortable shoes. If your shoes are tight or uncomfortable, all of you will be unhappy. Is the floor comfortable as well? If your feet rest on a hard, unyielding surface, the pressure will make them uncomfortable, especially if you take your shoes off when you type. If you have a carpet or pad to cushion the floor, that will take pressure off your feet. (Make sure that whatever you have under your feet does not create a high static electricity charge, which can damage your computer. If static electricity is a problem, there are products that allow you to ground yourself and discharge the static electricity before you touch your computer.)

INPUT DEVICES

Now that your chair and desk are adjusted correctly, we can turn our attention to the details of how your computer is set up. Let's start with input devices. For most people, the keyboard is the primary input device, followed perhaps by the mouse. Many people use trackballs instead of mice. Graphics (or digitizing) tablets are also frequently used. Telephones can be thought of as being part of the computer input process. In addition, with the adoption of voice recognition software, a microphone has also taken its place as an input device. We will examine body use for all of these devices.

KEYBOARD

The position and feel of your keyboard exert a lot of influence on how your fingers and hands are used. Though a few years back keyboards on personal computers were often not separate from the central processor and monitor, nowadays, as a general rule, desktop computers do have separate keyboards. This is important because it is necessary to position the keyboard and monitor independently in order to adjust the workstation to your particular physical requirements. (Laptops, however, do not have the three components separate, and we shall discuss this in Chapter 16.)

POSITIONING: How should you position your keyboard? Once you are sitting upright, with your desk and chair adjusted properly for your body, and with your hands out in front of you ready to type, the appropriate distance to your keyboard will become clear. The

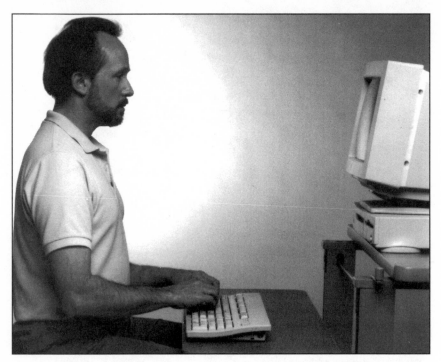

The correct distance to the keyboard allows the elbows to hang by the sides.

home row of keys (the ASDFG row on the QWERTY keyboard—the usual keyboard, which has the keys arranged so that the six keys at the left of the top alphabet row are in the order QWERTY) should fall right under your fingertips. You should not have to reach forward to get to the keyboard, nor should you have to pull back.

How far to the left or right should your keyboard be positioned? That depends on what you are typing. If you are using mostly or exclusively the alphabetic portion of the keyboard, the center of that section, rather than the center of the keyboard as a whole, should be right in front of the centerline of your body. On almost all keyboards, the cursor control keys and the number pad are at the right side. If you were to center the keyboard as a whole in front of you, the left edge of the alphabetic keys would be farther from your midline than the right edge would be, and you would have to twist to the left to place your fingers on the home keys. Aligning your body's center with the center of the alphabetic section of the keyboard allows you to position your hands and arms symmetrically and evenly as you type. If you are typing only on the number pad, you can position the keyboard so that the number pad falls directly under your typing hand (whether it is your left or right hand).

SLANT: The slant of the keyboard is also important. Most keyboards are higher in the rear, and consequently there is a downward slant to the key rows. For greatest comfort, your wrists and forearms should be straight as you type, but if the keyboard slopes upward significantly, you will most likely bend your wrists back to position your hands on the keyboard. Aside from the strain this puts on your wrists, it will encourage you to rest your wrists on the desk surface, and the pressure from this can irritate your wrists.

If your keyboard is slanted enough to be uncomfortable, this can be fixed easily. First, make sure that the legs at the rear of the keyboard are not extended. If the keyboard is still slanted too much, go to the hardware store and get some adhesive-backed foam weather strip tape and stick it under the front edge of the keyboard. You can use thin tape to raise the front just a bit or use layers of tape to make the keyboard perfectly level. This affects the thickness of the keyboard, and if you make a large change you might need to adjust your chair or desk.

Two other keyboard positions should be mentioned. I've experimented with having my keyboard slant away from me and with having it on my lap. Slanting it away presents problems. If you slant it away by raising the front edge of the keyboard, that large change will require that you raise your chair or lower the desk. If you don't, the keyboard will be too high. You can slant the keyboard away by lowering the rear edge, but of course that requires lowering the desk. Whether you lower your desk or raise your chair, you may not have enough leg room under your desk. If you are using an under-desk keyboard shelf, you could more easily slant the keyboard away from you, but that still might restrict your leg room. I haven't found slanting the keyboard away from me to be helpful, but you may wish to experiment with it and see whether it makes your shoulders, arms, wrists, and hands more comfortable.

Putting the keyboard on your lap is also problematic. Having your hands forward and down on your lap will drag your shoulders and neck forward and down. And it may be hard to balance the keyboard on your lap. If you use primarily the alphabetic keys, the keyboard has to be moved over to the right, and the left end won't sit securely on your left leg. To balance the keyboard on your lap, you may have to put it on a board. Of course, I am talking here about putting the keyboard on your lap as you sit in a centered position. If you recline, the same problems exist, and you add to it the problems of the reclining posture.

FEEL: The feel of your keyboard exerts a lot of influence on how you use your fingers and hands. If your keyboard has a stiff feel that makes you press each key down firmly, that will waste a lot of energy. If the keyboard makes the keys hit bottom with a hard contact, that will result in a lot of shock on your fingers and hands. Ideally, your keyboard should have a light, airy feel, and it should let the keys reach bottom with a pillowy feel. This kind of keyboard will allow your fingers to fly across the keys, contacting them in a very light and gentle manner, and it will provide a lot of cushioning for your fingers.

If your keys hit bottom uncomfortably hard, you can change that by using thin weather strip tape. (The idea of using foam to pad the keys comes from a book entitled *Repetitive Strain Injury*, by Emil Pascarelli and Deborah Quilter. They suggest using corn pads, but I like the feel of weather strip better. Their book focuses on treatment once RSI has occurred and has a lot of good information.) Cut squares of the foam tape to put on the keys, and then write the letters on the tape so you can find the keys. (The adhesive could be hard to clean off if you decide to remove the tape, so you might want to cover the keys with masking tape and stick the weather strip to the masking tape.)

A keyboard that has a light feel is important in using the half-turned hand position recommended in *Comfort at Your Computer.* You may find that when you press the return key you are applying pressure with the outer edge of your little finger, which is not the natural direction for force application with the finger. The more natural movement would be to apply force downward with the pad of the finger. If you have an especially stiff keyboard and hit your keys hard, this pressure along the edge of your finger may prove to be irritating. A softer keyboard would help, as would moving your whole hand over rather than just extending your little finger.

A keyboard with a very light touch demands greater sensitivity and lightness in your hands. People whose hands are tight will have much less sensitivity and will prefer harder keys so they can really *push* them and *feel* them. This hard work will increase these people's tension and decrease their sensitivity, which will reinforce their preference for harder keys. However, once you get used to a keyboard with a lighter touch, you will find it will allow your hands to stay relaxed as you work and will make your typing much more comfortable.

I remember typing on my IBM Selectric® typewriter. It had an extraordinarily comfortable feel to the keys. The keys seemed to have some sort of suction to them. Once you depressed the keys just a bit, they seemed to take over and depress themselves the rest of the way. It encouraged a very light touch and reduced the impact and pressure on the fingertips. I have never found a computer keyboard as comfortable as the Selectric keyboard.

V-SHAPED KEYBOARDS: Most people use the straight, single-piece QWERTY keyboard that has been standard for years. However, there are keyboard alternatives becoming available, and you may wish to try out some of these. One kind of keyboard that is commonly available has the alphabetic section split in the middle so the keyboard assumes a V-shape. The keyboard may have the keys arranged in an immovable V shape, or the keyboard may hinge and adjust to form anything from a straight line across (just like normal keyboards) to a pronounced V shape. The number pad and the function keys may be on a separate unit with a short cable which plugs into the side of the keyboard.

This kind of keyboard was designed to prevent people from bending their wrists sideways as they position their hands on the keys. Many people do this, and it is very stressful on the wrists (as was discussed in Chapter 7). If the keyboard allows the angle to be adjusted, then people can match the angle of the rows of keys to the inward angle of their forearms/hands. By using a keyboard that places the keys on an angle, people can straighten out their wrists and avoid side-bending of their hands. If the number pad is separate, people can move it to whichever side of the keyboard is most comfortable.

However, a V-shaped keyboard may be missing the mark. It is true that with a straight keyboard you will have to bend your wrists a bit, but you will probably be able to use a standard keyboard comfortably. It depends on how you type, how you bend your wrists, how much you bend your wrists, and how long you type. For most people the most significant element in lateral bending of the wrists is whether they hold their elbows out away from their sides (as was discussed in Chapter 7). If your elbows hang close to your sides and you have the rest of your workstation and posture arranged correctly, you will most likely not need to bend your wrists outward much to position your fingers on the keys.

If you bend your wrists just a slight bit and do it by gently lengthening the thumb side of your wrist rather than tensely shortening the little finger side, that will loosen rather than constrict your wrist, and it may be comfortable for you. If your wrists are comfortable with the time periods your spend keyboarding, then an ordinary keyboard is fine for you. However, if you find your forearms angling inward more than you would like, the adjustable split keyboard could be helpful to you. If you pay attention to how you feel as you type, you can evaluate this for yourself.

By the way, does all this analysis of keyboard possibilities seem like an awful lot of attention to pay to such small details? Well, many people hurt themselves doing simple, every-day activities. If you are going to use your computer extensively, it is worth spending some time on doing so safely. Posture and movement are composed of nothing but details. If you are uncomfortable in some particular situation, this is the kind of detail thinking and exploration that will help you come up with a solution.

WRIST SUPPORTS

Wrist supports are used with keyboards, so now is a good time to discuss them. Should you use wrist supports to help support the weight of your arms as you type? This is really part of the question of what overall posture to sit in. If you are sitting in the reclining posture (see Chapter 11), you will have to hold your arms out in front of your body to reach your keyboard. In that position, the weight of your whole arm pulls down on your shoulders and chest. Wrist supports are not the solution, however. Wrist supports hold up only the wrist end of your arm. If you sit with your arms held out forward and your wrists on a wrist support, you will be able to feel that the weight of your upper arms still drags your chest and shoulders forward and down.

If you are sitting in either the straight up position or the centered position, your upper arms are down by your sides, so wrist rests will have to support just the weight of your forearms. In the straight up position, there will be tension in your chest, back, and shoulders. Since wrist rests won't relieve that, they won't improve the straight up sitting style significantly.

The centered position is still the best sitting position, and the question is whether a wrist support will improve it. My experience is that when I rest my arms on a wrist support, my hands and arms are less free to move around. I find this uncomfortable, and it violates a cardinal rule, which is to keep moving. In addition, keeping my wrists resting on the wrist rest forces me to confine my typing movements to my hands rather than using my whole arms. That violates another cardinal rule, which is to aid smaller muscles in their work by using larger muscles. Beyond that, the pressure on the underside of my wrists is also uncomfortable, and I imagine it could be very irritating in the long run. Again, I have to go back to the idea that the body is an elegant, self-supporting mechanism. If you use your body correctly, you will not find wrist supports comfortable or helpful.

MOUSE

With the advent of the Macintosh computer, the mouse became a major input device, and with the introduction of Windows, even more people adopted these little rodents. There are a number of issues to think about in comfortable mousing.

MOUSE POSITION: How you use your mouse arm will be greatly affected by the placement of your mouse. Should you put your mouse on the right or left side of your keyboard?

The number pad and cursor control keys are usually on the right side of the keyboard, and that means that when the alphabetic section is centered in front of you, the right end of the keyboard is about six inches (about fifteen centimeters) further from your body's centerline than is the left end. Most people are right-handed and place the mouse to the right of the keyboard. Notice that if you do so, you will have to hold your arm considerably farther away from your side than if you place your mouse to the left of your keyboard. That extra extension of your arm will result in significant fatigue and strain in your shoulder and neck. It could even affect your back.

It is a good idea to put the mouse on the left side of the keyboard—even though for right-handed people it takes getting used to. It may feel awkward at first, but you will get used to it soon, and you will find that it will considerably lessen the work your arm has to do in using the mouse. (This recommendation is for work involving text. If you do primarily graphics work, you may want a different mouse placement. See the section on Graphics Tablets and Drawing.)

HAND USE: How you use your hand on the mouse is important too. The anatomically normal position for a relaxed hand is with the fingers semi-curled, and that is just the position which most mice are designed to allow. Let your hand and fingers assume a comfortable, relaxed position around the mouse. Don't grip the mouse hard, and don't push down hard on the button. Consciously relax your hand as you use the mouse.

Some mice force you to bend your hand back a bit to use them, which puts a strain on the wrist and hand. In addition, it puts the rounded undersurface of your wrist lower than your hand on the mouse, and there will be a temptation to rest your wrist on the desk surface as you maneuver your mouse. That pressure and friction could lead to significant irritation as you use the mouse. To prevent that, hold your arm up a bit as you slide the mouse around your desk. You don't have to lift your hand high off the desk, but make sure to lift it enough to lessen the pressure.

If you let your arm press onto the edge of the desk as you use your mouse, that will be much more irritating and dangerous than simple pressure on the desk surface. Stay aware and don't adopt lazy habits of movement. Keep the pressure off the underside of your arm.

MOUSE FEEL: Just as with the keyboard itself, the feel of the mouse and the buttons on the mouse will be important. The mouse should be light and easy to move, and the buttons should be light enough that they don't take significant force to push down. Compared to the mouse I got when I first started using a computer, many new mice are considerably lighter, are shaped more smoothly for the hand, and have buttons that are larger and easier to push. The changes add up to a mouse that is more comfortable to use and worth buying as a replacement for the older mice.

TRACKBALL

Many people use trackballs instead of mice. Trackballs are essentially mice on their backs. With a mouse, you move the whole mouse in order to roll the ball on its underside against the desk surface. With a trackball, the ball is on top, and you move it directly with one or two fingers. Since a trackball stays stationary on the desk, it takes less effort than a mouse to use. It does not require you to move your whole arm, and you can keep your arm close to the side of your keyboard. Just as with a mouse, the trackball should be placed to the left of your keyboard for ordinary alphabetic typing.

Since you don't have to move your whole arm to use a trackball, you may find yourself doing all the trackball movements with just your fingers/hand/wrist. That could put quite a strain on your wrist. You may also find yourself bending your hand backwards to position it on the trackball, especially if the trackball is thick and large. That would create more strain on your wrist. Be careful to keep your hand in a neutral, comfortable position as you use your trackball. Use your whole arm even for the small movements the trackball requires.

The feel of the trackball buttons and the movements required for using the trackball must be comfortable for to make using it worthwhile. Trackballs will be most comfortable if the buttons are so light that they don't take significant force to push down. Some trackballs require that you push a button with the side of your thumb. If you think about it, you will realize that the thumb is built for pinching movements using the pad of the thumb. It is not built for exerting significant strength or pressure with the side of the thumb. I used one common trackball for a while that had very firm buttons and required pressing a button with the side of the thumb. At first it felt quite comfortable because of the greater efficiency of movement, but very soon my hand and thumb became quite sore, and I stopped using the trackball.

There are many different styles of trackballs, and you could experiment with them to find one that works well for you. Try various trackballs to find one that it fits your hand comfortably. Make sure that you try out each one for a long enough period of time to really feel how it will affect your movements during long work hours.

GRAPHICS TABLETS, DRAWING, AND HANDWRITING RECOGNITION

OK. Here we go. This will be an adventure. This section is about the use of graphics (digitizing) tablets, and I am writing it on a tablet that includes handwriting recognition software.

Tablets are flat writing surfaces, generally about the size of paper notebooks and about a quarter-inch thick (about six-tenths of a centimeter). They have special pens, and whatever shapes are traced on the tablet appear on the screen. Many artists use digitizing tablets for drawing because they allow people who are used to pen and ink to draw in their familiar ways and yet still work on computers.

It is also possible to draw using a mouse. As the mouse is rolled around the desk, the path it follows shows up as a line on the computer screen. Even though this section is about graphics tablets, it will include some information about drawing with a mouse since the movements of using a mouse or tablet are so similar.

The tablet I am using is the Handwriter, from Communication Intelligence Corporation. It comes with handwriting recognition software, so it is capable of handling alphanumeric data input as well as drawing.

I must say that it is strange to be writing into my computer. I type faster than I write, and certainly more neatly. For twenty-five years I have typed every article, story, or paper I have written, and for the last ten years I have been doing all my typing on a computer.

The first thing that I have to get used to is that graphics tablets, unlike mice, are absolute indicators of position. Each point on the tablet corresponds to one point on the screen. With a mouse, the cursor moves only when the mouse rolls across the desk surface. When the mouse is held in the air, moving it doesn't affect the position of the cursor. But with a graphics tablet, if the pen is picked up and moved two inches over, the cursor will appear two inches from where it had been when the pen was lifted. If a circle is drawn on the lower right corner of the tablet, it will appear on the lower right corner of the screen.

I also have to get used to the fact that some care is needed to print in the neat style this software needs for optimal handwriting recognition. And it is necessary to learn the marks this software uses for editing. However, none of that is difficult, and as I work with Handwriter, it is becoming easier and faster to use.

Handwriting recognition does take some getting used to, and if you are a good typist, you may find it slower than a keyboard. However, it could be a viable keyboard replacement or supplement. Individuals who do not know how to type well or who are physically incapable of using a keyboard could find it valuable. It also allows people to work at a computer using very different hand movements, which could be helpful in reducing muscular fatigue and strain from keyboarding.

Whether a tablet is used for graphics or text, using one is like writing or drawing on paper. You move your hand across the tablet surface to write across or draw on the computer screen. However, even the ordinary movements of drawing or writing can be fatiguing and injurious. Down through the centuries, writers have suffered from writer's cramp and hand injuries.

It is important to sit and move properly to maintain comfort and avoid strain when using digitizing tablets. The first thing to think about is positioning. Where do you put the tablet for greatest comfort? How do you position your body as a whole and your arm and hand in particular?

TABLET POSITION: To begin with, let's consider the overall body positioning required. Using a tablet is very unlike writing in that nothing you draw on the tablet shows up on the tablet. Instead, you must keep your eyes focused on the computer screen, which is where anything you draw will show up. Since you must sit facing the monitor squarely to see the screen without twisting your body, the best position for the monitor will be on the desk straight in front of you. (See the discussion on monitor placement later in this chapter.)

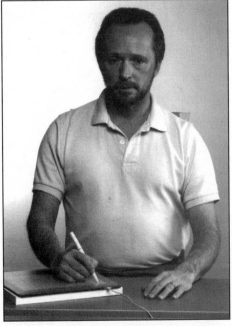

Position the graphics tablet to the side and somewhat slanted. Place it on a thin book if the desk height is adjusted for keyboarding.

Since you must sit facing the monitor, you will be in essentially the same position as when using a keyboard, and all of the rules for balanced sitting still apply. You should maintain an erect sitting posture. Your feet should be flat on the floor with your knees spread comfortably apart.

The tablet itself should be on your desk off to one side of your body. If you write with your right hand, the tablet should be to your right. Sit in the centered position, with your right elbow hanging naturally by your side and your right hand on your desk. Place the center of the tablet in front of your elbow. Position the tablet at a distance that allows your hand to rest naturally about halfway between the top and bottom edges of the drawing area. Now move the tablet straight to your left just a bit, and tilt the tablet to move the upper left corner of the tablet just a little bit more to left.

Why should this placement be comfortable? It has to do with the movement of the hand across the surface of the tablet. Let your elbow hang comfortably by your side, put your right hand on your desk and move your hand back and forth, left and right. Notice that the right-left movements of your hand describe an arc, with the bone in your upper arm (the humerus) being the center of the circle of which the arc is a piece. The construction of the shoulder girdle does not allow your hand to arc as far to the right as to the left, so the midpoint of the arc is closer to your body. A left-to-right stoke starts in toward your body's midline, moves up and out to the right, reaches the top of the arc, and then finishes just about in front of the humerus. The placement of the tablet that I recommended is the best fit for the natural side-to-side movement of the hand. If you positioned the tablet square on your desk instead of at a slight angle, that would demand a little bit more work from your shoulder.

When they write, many people position the paper so that it is much farther to their left and much more slanted toward the left (again, talking about right handed people). Then they twist their bodies and angle their arms to position their hands for writing. That creates a good deal of strain, and a more open body use will be much more comfortable. Left-handed people should also experiment with opening their body and arm use and sitting more square to the desk.

DESK HEIGHT: The desk height should be such that your elbow is held at about a right angle as your writing hand rests on the tablet.

A graphics tablet is thinner than a keyboard, and although the difference is minimal, that height difference does affect arm position a bit and therefore desk height. (See the discussion earlier in this chapter on desk height for writing.) If your desk height is set for keyboard use, you might find that there will be a slight strain on the shoulder of your writing/drawing hand from holding your hand just a bit too low down. If so, the easy way to solve that—presuming you want to be able to use both a keyboard and tablet—is to put a half-inch thick book under the tablet to raise it up to keyboard height. Make sure that your desk is not so high that the underside of your forearm presses against the edge of the graphics tablet as you draw on it.

KEYBOARD PLACEMENT: You will still find a keyboard useful while you are using a graphics tablet. Even with Handwriter, which allows the equivalent of keyboard command key functions using the tablet pen, it is still more convenient to do some things directly on the keyboard. If you are using a graphics tablet that does not include handwriting recognition software, then you will of course need a keyboard for ordinary alphanumeric input. You can experiment with positioning your keyboard off to the left of your tablet (assuming again that you are right handed), but that will require you to twist to the left to use the keyboard. Or you can place the keyboard behind the tablet, in front of your monitor, but that will require you to lean forward. Both options will result in some strain, but you may have no choice, and you will simply have to do the movements as efficiently as possible.

Whichever movement you choose, remember to use your whole body to do it. If you elect to twist to the side, start the movement by pushing down on the floor with your right foot, and let the movement travel up your leg and through your pelvis into your torso. (See Movement #5 of the Spiral Movements exercise in Chapter 12.) If you elect to lean forward, make sure you lean from your hip sockets rather than bending your back. (See the Airport Duck exercise in Chapter 8.)

HAND USE: Just as in ordinary writing, and unlike in keyboarding, all the work is done with just one hand. This means that you will have to do something with the hand that is not using the pen, and you will probably be most comfortable with it on the desk in front of you. Make sure that you relax your idle hand and position it comfortably while using a tablet. If you fail to keep that hand comfortable, your whole body will be affected.

Just as in ordinary writing, it is very easy to grip the pen too hard or press down too hard on the tablet. Many people tense their faces or mouths as they write. Watch out for tension and effort as you use a digitizing tablet. Continue to pay attention to how your body feels as you write or draw. Relax, breathe easily and search for balance in your body.

BODY TENSION: Be especially careful of eye strain and whole body tension that comes from writing on the tablet but keeping an unbroken visual focus on the screen. Normally we see what we write or draw on the paper as we do it. If you grip the screen with your eyes, watching for a visible result of the movements you are making on the tablet, you will tend to slip into a rigid, strained position of unbroken concentration. You may find yourself staring unblinkingly at the screen. Keep blinking and keep moving.

Some people lean back in their chairs and put the tablet on their laps, but if you pay attention to how you feel working with the tablet on your lap, you will notice the same postural compression and strain that we discussed in the section on the reclining posture (in Chapter 11). However, even a position that you may not wish to stay in for very long can be useful as a change from an overall better working posture.

DRAWING WITH A MOUSE: The process of drawing with a mouse is nearly identical to the process of drawing on a graphics tablet. Instead of drawing on the area defined by the tablet, the mouse moves across an equivalent clear space on the desk. Since the arm movements will be the same, the clear desk space should be in the same location that the tablet would occupy. The same requirements for keyboard placement still apply. (In the section on using a mouse, I recommended placing it to the left of your keyboard. Naturally that was for keyboard-focused operations, not drawing. And of course, for drawing you will be using your preferred hand.)

There is one major difference, and that is hand use. Holding a pen allows the hand to assume a very natural and comfortable half-turned position. Placing the hand in the fairly flat position necessary for using the mouse is not as comfortable for drawing. In particular, when you use a mouse to draw, you have to hold down the button to draw a line, and that constant action of pressing down can produce a lot of strain. That strain will tense your whole body. Make sure to take rest and movement breaks to relieve the strain. You can also buy a mouse or trackball that will keep the button held down after you click it until you click it a second time. That will prevent a lot of strain.

TELEPHONE

A telephone is an input device, in a manner of speaking. For some people the telephone is the source of the information they enter into their computers. If you need to use both hands for typing, you may find yourself scrunching up your shoulder to hold the telephone hand piece in position by your ear (even if the hand piece has a cradle attached to its back). Over any length of time, this will result in severe strain. Using a headset telephone will allow you to wear an earpiece and a mouthpiece instead of holding a hand piece, and that will enable you to maintain a normal, comfortable head and neck position as you talk on the phone.

VOICE RECOGNITION

Voice recognition software uses a microphone to input speech to the computer and software to translate that speech into text. Aside from the important requirement of not straining when you speak, there is little that needs to be said about voice recognition. Since the microphones are generally in a headset, like a telephone headset, they don't lead to any postural strain.

MACROS

Though a macro is not an input device, a brief mention of the use of macros is relevant here. Macros are simple scripts of instructions that you set up either in the main applications you use or with specific macro software. If you do tasks which contain repetitious keyboarding, you can automate them with macros. You can save time and keystrokes and greatly reduce the work your hands and fingers have to do by having the computer do whole sequences of actions with just one keystroke. Whatever input devices you use, macros will allow you to use them less.

MONITOR

Your monitor affects your comfort in two ways. The technical characteristics of the monitor determine how comfortable it will be to look at, and the positioning of the monitor is a major factor in determining how comfortable your posture will be.

Technical Characteristics of the Monitor

The technical characteristics of the monitor determine the quality of the visual images produced. Characteristics of the text display also affect your visual comfort and will be discussed here.

MONITOR: For the common cathode ray tube monitor, the image you see is painted onto your monitor in horizontal lines, the same way a television works. The screen on a desktop monitor is coated inside with chemicals that glow when they are hit by electrons from the electron guns at the back of the cathode ray tube (CRT). The computer breaks down an image into a series of dots located along the horizontal lines on the screen. The electron guns sweep along those lines, either turning on dots (pixels) or passing over them. By moving over the whole screen very rapidly, the electron guns assemble enough glowing dots to create a picture. Although the screen really shows nothing but lines of dots, they are painted on more rapidly than the eye and brain can detect, so they are perceived as solid images. (Screens on laptops work in a similar manner, but they don't use an electron gun to turn on the dots on the screen. The new, flat monitors which are becoming available for desktop computers work the same way laptop screens do.)

The image you are looking at should be well-focused. The electron guns in the CRT should be able to focus sharply and turn on just the dots required for an image. This is particularly important with color monitors, which have three streams of electrons to focus together. The range of colors you see on the monitor is assembled by turning on dots in the three basic colors of red, green, and blue. Each color is controlled by one gun, and if the three guns do not converge correctly, images will be fuzzy.

Your monitor should produce clear, sharp images. It should have good contrast between the image and the screen background. Contrast will be enhanced by having smaller screen dots, which will produce finer detail in the image. Having dark text characters on a light background (rather than vice versa) will enhance contrast, as will minimizing glare. Having a screen which can be adjusted to a sufficient brightness will enhance your visual comfort, both directly by providing images that are easy to look at, and indirectly by overcoming glare. The screen should be uniformly bright everywhere rather than having variations in different spots.

Sharpness will also be improved by dusting off your screen. Because of the electrostatic charge of your screen, it will actually attract dust particles, which will coat the screen and degrade the image quality. Dust your screen frequently. (Make sure to use something that will not scratch the surface of your screen. Different screens have different surfaces, so you may want to check on what would be safe for your particular screen.)

The images on your screen should be stable and correctly proportioned. They should not jitter or drift around. And your monitor should produce straight lines that are actually straight, rather than bent somewhat. Some monitors have controls to adjust the straightness of their lines.

Some screens are roughened or coated to reduce reflections or glare, and some people use glare reduction filters over the monitor. Such treatments can reduce glare, but make sure that they don't also reduce sharpness to an unacceptable extent.

Keep these technical characteristics in mind as you examine the monitor you use or any monitor you are considering buying. The basic idea is that lines and characters should be sharp and clear on the edges, which will make them a lot more comfortable to look at.

TEXT: The visual qualities of the text displayed on your monitor directly affect your visual comfort. To begin with, the point size of your text is related to your visual needs and the distance you sit from your monitor. If you sit farther back from the screen to reduce stress on your eyes (see Chapter 10), you may need to increase the point size of your text to see it comfortably. Is the job you are doing designed in such a way that you can change the size of the text to fit your needs or are you stuck with a one-size-fits-all display? If you are using a database or spreadsheet, your screen display may have been designed with certain text sizes required to fit information into certain boxes. If you are preparing simple text such as journal articles or business letters, you may more easily be able to change font size. If you can change the text size, experiment with different sizes until you discover what is most comfortable for you. Some applications allow you to change the size of the screen image independent of the actual font size.

You should choose the fonts themselves for greatest ease and comfort in reading. Note that what is comfortable to look at and easy to read on the monitor may not be what is best on a printed page. Choose a font that is comfortable for screen use, and if there is a conflict between visual comfort in reading a screen and desired appearance on the final printed page, you can always compose your text in one font or one size and then change it for layout and printing.

There are many elements that go into font design. The weight of the lines that form the characters, the size and shape of the characters, the space between the characters, and the space between lines all contribute to the visual feel of a font. For large blocks of text, text with both upper and lower case letters is easier to read. Larger font sizes are easier to see, but if the font size is too large, you will be able to see fewer words at a time, which will make the text harder to read.

Experiment with the appearance of your fonts, and try to find text that is visually comfortable and satisfying to look at. There is a lot of material available in the areas of typography and visual design, and there is much more to learn about this if it interests you.

RADIATION: Radiation is a technical characteristic of monitors that should be mentioned, although it doesn't have a direct effect on your comfort at your workstation. There is a lot of debate about whether radiation from monitors has damaging effects. Speaking very conservatively, it can't hurt to minimize the radiation you receive. If it turns out that the effects of radiation are really unimportant, then the money or effort expended on reducing radiation will have been wasted. However, that may be unimportant compared to the possibility of preventing radiation damage in case it is discovered that radiation from monitors is truly injurious.

The simplest way to cut down on radiation is to move the monitor father away from you. The inverse square law states that the amount of radiation received from a radiation source decreases as the square of the distance from the source. That means that if you double the distance from the monitor you receive one quarter the radiation. By sitting an arm's length or more from an average monitor, you reduce your radiation exposure to low levels.

It is also important not to sit beside or behind monitors. The greatest amount of radiation comes from the back and sides of the monitor. Your workstation may have an area beside or behind your monitor where you spend a good deal of time, or you may be near someone else's monitor. Think about whether you are sitting immediately behind a monitor in the next office. Even if there is a wall between you and the monitor, you may still receive significant radiation. If you leave five feet or so (one and a half meters) between you and other computers, you will be much safer. You may also wish to turn off your monitor when you are not using it. That will reduce your exposure to radiation, and it will have the environmental benefit of conserving energy.

Aside from proper positioning, another way to cut down on radiation is to buy monitors that emit less radiation. There are standards for radiation emission that have international acceptance. Check for compliance with these standards when you buy new monitors. Older monitors may not have been designed with radiation standards in mind. A third way to reduce radiation is to buy radiation shields. Depending on the shield, these may cut down radiation emitted in different directions by your monitor.

For current information on monitor quality and radiation emissions, the best source is articles in the various computer magazines.

Positioning the Monitor

How far from you should you place your monitor? How high or low should it be? And should it be in front of you or to the side? The position of your monitor is determined by the position of your body and by how your eyes work.

DIRECTION: Sit upright in the centered position. Make sure your head and eyes are in their place of balance and comfort, and then place your monitor where your eyes point. Since your eyes point forward, your monitor should be placed in front of you.

I've often seen people position their keyboards right in front of them and their monitors to the side—usually because their desks are to narrow to allow them to place their monitors directly in front. Placing the monitor to the side forces you to twist yourself to the side, which is very unbalanced and creates a good deal of strain over

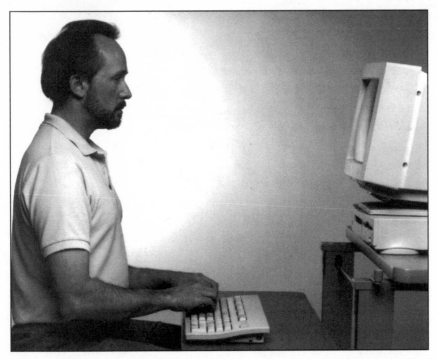

The monitor should be about an arm's length away and tilted to meet the angle of the eyes.

any lengthy period of work. If your desk is too narrow and it is right up against the wall, you may be able to get more space for your monitor simply by moving your desk away from the wall.

DISTANCE: Think about sitting in a movie theater. The farther away you sit from the screen, the smaller the screen seems to be. That is, it takes up a smaller percentage of your total field of vision. If your monitor is very close to your eyes, it will subsume a large angle in your field of vision. In that case, if you position the top of your monitor where you find it comfortable to look, you will have to shift your eyes quite a distance down to look at the bottom of the screen. Or you will have to tilt your head down to look at the bottom of the screen. Either alternative will result in excess muscle use and undue fatigue.

How far away from you should your monitor be? Remember that the resting focal distance for the eyes is around 32 inches (81 centimeters) for an adult. If you have good vision, normal or corrected with glasses, you will probably find that you will be most comfortable looking at a monitor which is placed an arm's length or a bit more from you. (The resting focal distance may be somewhat shorter for a child, but having children place the monitor at their arm's length or a bit more is still about right.) That will help you avoid the extra effort that close visual focus requires of your eye muscles. In addition, moving your monitor that far away means it subsumes a smaller visual angle, and your eyes won't have to travel as far to look from the top of the screen to the bottom or from side to side. For both those reasons, keeping your monitor at about an arm's length will be more efficient and more comfortable. Of course, that means that your desk has to be wide enough to accommodate that distance.

HEIGHT AND ANGLE: How high or low should your monitor be? The natural line of gaze for your eyes is about ten to fifteen degrees below horizontal, so your monitor placement should allow that downward line of vision. Your eyes should rest naturally on the middle of your screen. It takes work (in both your eyes and your neck) to look up or down, and the farther up or down you look, the more work it takes. If your monitor is positioned so that your gaze falls on the middle of your screen, then you will be moving your eyes about the same amount upward to the top of the screen and downward to the bottom, which will be most efficient. For an average size monitor, if you place the top of your screen (not the top of your monitor, but the top of the image area) about level with your eyes, that will put the middle of your screen at about the right place. Of course, if you have a very large monitor, this formula may not be quite right.

Notice that if your gaze is angled downward and your monitor's face is vertical, you will be viewing your monitor at an angle rather than straight on. In order to have your monitor meet your gaze most comfortably, you will want the monitor tilted up a bit so that its face is perpendicular to your line of sight.

MONITOR STAND: What do you put your monitor on? How can you adjust its height and angle to meet your visual needs? How do you have your monitor positioned now? Very often people place their monitor on top of their central processing unit (the actual computer itself, abbreviated CPU), and possibly on top of an external hard disk as well. This arrangement is convenient in terms of saving desk space, but it may not put the monitor at the appropriate height or angle.

For some computers, the monitor and CPU are all one piece, and that means positioning your whole computer according to where you need your monitor to be. On most computers, the monitor and CPU are separate, and the monitor can be positioned separately. Many monitors have a built in tilt/swivel stand, which eases the job of positioning the monitor at the right angle. However, tilt/swivel stands generally do not include a way of adjusting monitor height, so even a monitor with a tilt stand will probably still need to be on a support of some kind. There are desks and monitor supports commercially available that allow you to move your monitor up and down and vary its tilt as well. (See the Resources section at the end of this chapter.)

One simple way to support the monitor in the right position is to build a stand for it. In the following discussion, I will assume you are going to build a stand for a monitor that lacks a tilt/swivel stand. If you have a commercial monitor stand that allows both height and angle adjustments, the process of finding the right monitor placement will be much the same.

Experiment with your monitor height and angle until you discover what is most comfortable. Start by stacking up a bunch of thin books or sheets of plywood to put your monitor on. Make sure that the stack is *stable* and *strong*. You don't want your monitor to crash to the floor. When you place your monitor on the stack of books, put something under the front of the monitor to tilt it up toward your face. That could be a rolled up section of newspaper or a piece of wood.

Make the stack higher than you could possibly want your monitor to be. Then sit and work at your computer. Feel how your body responds to working with the monitor at that height. Experiment a bit with the angle of tilt of the monitor to find the most comfortable angle for that height.

Then slip out one book and try working with the monitor at a slightly lower height. Keep reducing the stack height until the monitor is clearly too low, feeling how your body responds at each height. At each height, experiment with the tilt of the monitor. Go back and forth until you feel clearly the most comfortable height and monitor angle. That is the positioning you need, and your stand should support your monitor in that position.

A monitor stand can easily be made out of inch thick plywood (about two and half centimeters). You can build a shelf that will support your monitor at the right height. A piece of wood nailed to the front edge of shelf will serve to raise the front of the monitor and tilt it to the angle you need. I would suggest making the stand open in the front and back, which would allow you to run your cables through. And if you make your stand a bit wider than your keyboard, having the front open allows you to slide your keyboard under your monitor and out of the way. That can be convenient when you need extra desk space for non-computer work.

This stand is non-adjustable, but it is adjusted precisely to your needs. Of course, as you continue to pay attention to your body and improve your posture, your needs or your perception of your needs may change, and you might have to rebuild the stand. If you are sharing your computer with co-workers, or perhaps with the rest of your family, you will need an adjustable setup, and an adjustable commercial support may be best.

LOCATION: Where in the room should you locate your desk and monitor? How do you have them positioned now? Is the back of your monitor up against a blank wall? If so, then you will be able to look only from your monitor to the wall, which doesn't offer much change of visual focus. Remember that close focus is more fatiguing to your eyes. Ideally you should position your monitor so you can look out of a window, off into the distance for a few seconds every ten minutes or so. (Remember, however, not to position your computer so that backlighting from the window results in glare.) If is not possible to have a view out a window, you should at least be able to look across the room or down a hallway.

If your monitor is placed against a wall and you don't have a window to look through, you can still look off into the distance by placing a mirror on the wall in front of you. (The idea of putting a mirror by the desk comes from *Total Health at the Computer*, by Sussman, Lowenstein, and Sann. It is such a good idea that I felt I had to mention it, but contrary to the title, the book is primarily about an approach to eye care and has only a superficial treatment of overall body use.) Though the mirror is on the wall in front of you, your eyes will focus as though they were looking across the whole distance of the room behind you. You can feel the way this works by first focusing on the glass of the mirror and then looking *into* the mirror and focusing on the image there. In fact this makes a good eye exercise.

PAPER DOCUMENTS

Your computer work may involve using books or other paper documents, both for reading from and writing on. Your head movements, visual refocusing, body position, and body use are influenced by what documents you need to look at, where they are placed, and what you have to do with them.

READ ONLY DOCUMENT POSITIONS: There are a number of positions you can use for read only paper documents: (1) flat on the desk beside the keyboard, (2) flat in front of you between the keyboard and the monitor, (3) propped up at an angle to the side and in front of the monitor, or (4) propped up at an angle in front of you between the keyboard and the monitor. Each of these positions will involve different head, eye, and body use.

There are two movements that can be involved in looking from your screen to your paper documents and back again—nodding your head up and down, and turning your head from side to side. Doing either of these movements means moving your head off the vertical, balanced position of efficient support and comfort, and doing either of these movements over a long period of computer use will produce fatigue and strain. Placing your documents properly will minimize these movements and the resulting fatigue as much as possible.

What document positions will be best? To start with, you should avoid placing your paper documents flat on your desk. To see them you would have to drop your head forward and down, a position that would be very fatiguing to maintain. Just as the screen should be tilted to meet the line of your gaze, so too should documents be tilted.

If you position your documents at the same height as your screen, you will have to position them next to the screen and turn your head back and forth from the screen to the documents. This will reduce the up and down movements of your head and eyes but increase the side to side movements. If you do position documents to the side of your screen, make sure to periodically switch the side you use. If you keep the documents on the same side all the time, you will be using the same muscles in the same orientation for long periods, which will create fatigue and strain.

If you prop up your read only documents in front of you between your keyboard and screen, that will minimize the side to side movements of your head but require more up and down movements.

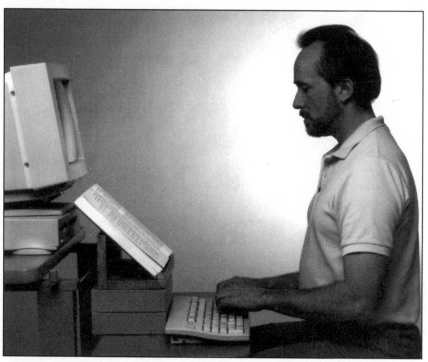

One way of positioning and supporting paper documents.

Tilting your head forward and down to look down means moving the weight of your head forward, off its base of support. In that position, your muscles must work hard to support your head. In side-to-side movements, the weight of your head stays balanced on its base of support, and your head is simply swiveled left and right. For that reason, you may find up and down head movements to be more fatiguing than side-to-side movements.

However, the higher you position your documents, the less you will need to bend your head forward. Since your screen will be fairly high off the desk to meet the line of your gaze, that will allow enough room to prop up even good-sized books in front of you without their getting in the way of your screen. You may find that propping books up in front of you will offer the best trade-off between bending and rotating movements. On the other hand, if your documents are too large, they will have to be positioned to the side, and they should then be as close as possible to the screen to minimize turning movements.

Try positioning the documents beside or in front of the screen to discover what is most comfortable for you. You might find that different documents and different tasks are most comfortable in different positions. You might also find that placing documents alternately in front of and beside the screen allows you to increase the variety of your movements and reduce the fatigue of spending long periods in one position.

What documents you use will determine what you need to hold them up. You may be using small or large sheets of paper, single sheets, stacks of paper, or bound books. The simplest and most flexible document holder is a stand that will prop up on an angle the wide variety of documents you may use. There are commercial document stands and clips for supporting various documents in various positions. Or you can easily build a document stand. Nail two six inch (fifteen centimeter) wide boards together to form an L-shape, and then nail an eighth-inch (three-tenths of a centimeter) strip of wood down the front edge of the bottom board to keep documents from slipping off. The exact document angle that will be most comfortable for you depends on your height, so you may want the back board of the stand to be a bit more or less than six inches wide.

A very simple way to support documents is to roll up a towel and place it behind the document. You can leave a bit of towel unrolled to place the bottom edge of the document on. That will keep the document from sliding off the towel. If you are using a book on a document holder, you may find the pages flipping themselves rather than laying open to the spot you want. A simple solution to this is to keep a length of light chain handy and drape it across the pages to keep them flat.

LIGHTING: In addition to the position of the documents, how you light them is also important. If you use spot lighting on your documents and they are much brighter than your screen, your eyes will have to adapt to different levels of illumination every time you shift your focus back and forth from screen to document. On the other hand, if your documents are not illuminated brightly enough, you may experience discomfort from that as well. Try different levels of illumination on the documents along with different levels of screen brightness and room illumination until you find what is most comfortable for you. Sometimes you will find that overhead lights provide good illumination but shine in your eyes. A simple solution is to wear a visor to shade your eyes.

WRITE AND READ DOCUMENTS: If you have to write on your paper documents, you will have to place them next to your keyboard simply to reach them, and the documents can either lie flat on your desk or be propped up at a shallow angle on a writing stand. The placement of write-on documents will require looking down at the paper and up at the screen, so it will be important to move your head in a balanced, efficient way and take frequent rest or movement breaks.

If you rarely use your keyboard but do quite a bit of writing, you can put the documents on your desk immediately in front of you with the keyboard behind the document. You will have to reach across the documents to your keyboard, but that may be acceptable if you need to do it infrequently.

Positioning write-on documents can get complicated. There are a number of variables. Are you right or left handed? Do you do most of your work on the alphabetic keys or on the numeric keypad? Does your keyboard allow you to switch the keypad from right to left so that it can be positioned for easy use with your favored hand, or moved out of the way if you don't use it much? Do you have a separate numeric keypad, which would allow you to move your keyboard out of the way if you don't use it at all?

If you are right handed, you will want the paper on the right of your keyboard. However, if you use the alphabetic keys and cannot reposition the numeric keypad, that will place the paper rather far out to your right. You may be forced to keep moving the keyboard and the paper back and forth to get each positioned for comfortable use. However, if you use only the numeric keypad, you can position the keypad close to the midline of your body and the paper document to the right of the keypad, close to you. Remember the description in the section on Graphics Tablets of the arc movements of the hand? Since the hand will move in an arc from left to right between the keypad and the paper, you may want to angle your keyboard a bit to the left and the paper a bit to the right as they rest on the desk. That will allow a natural placement of your hand as you turn to each.

If you are left handed, and if you are using primarily the numeric keypad and writing on paper, you can move the keyboard far to the left and have the paper roughly in front of you. Of course, you will also have to figure out where to put your mouse. But if you are using both the alphabetic keys and a mouse along with write-on paper documents, where do you put all those things?

Well, I'm not even going to try to deal with every possible combination of situations. It would be ideal if the numeric keypad and the alphabetic keys were detachable so they could be arranged on your desk to suit your handedness and the tasks you have to do. You could use a swivel chair and arrange the different documents and the monitor and keyboard so that you can turn from one to the other as you work.

If you have to write on paper documents, however you arrange your work, keep in mind the principles of balanced relaxed body use and experiment with different setups until you find one that is comfortable. Try to keep everything you work with in front of you and as close to your body's centerline as possible. Try to use both hands as evenly as possible. And pay attention to using your whole body in comfortable ways as you write and type.

RESOURCES

There is a lot of material in the field of ergonomics and office design. With the exception of some aspects of the work done on body use and sitting, much of it is valuable for people concerned with computer use. Two good books are:

Ergonomics in Computerized Offices. Etienne Grandjean. Taylor & Francis, London, 1987.

Ergonomics, Work and Health. Stephen Pheasant. Aspen Publishers, Gaithersburg, Maryland. 1991.

The very first ergonomics text was published over two hundred years ago, and it is fascinating to read:

Diseases of Workers. Bernardino Ramazzini. Translated by Wilmer Cave Wright from the Latin text *De Morbis Artificum*, of 1713. Hafner Publishing Company, New York, 1964.

There is a lot of ergonomically oriented office equipment available commercially. Much of it is based on fallacious ideas of how to use the body, but a lot of the equipment—monitor supports, desk risers, keyboard shelves, document stands, and so on—can be helpful. Two useful catalogs are:

AliMed, Ergonomics and Occupational Health Catalog. 297 High Street, Dedham, MA 02026, USA. Phone 800-225-2610. Fax 617-329-8392. http://www.alimed.com.

Global Computer Supplies. 2249 Windsor Court, Addison, IL 60101, USA. Phone 800-845-6225. Fax 708-627-1742. http://www.global-computer.com.

There are websites and newslists devoted to various aspects of computer use and Repetitive Strain Injuries. Two useful resources are:

SOREHAND is a newslist with an accompanying website. You can subscribe from the website, which is at http://www.ucsf.edu/sorehand.

TIFAQ (typing injury—frequently asked questions) is a website at http://www.tifaq.org.

KEY POINTS

- Experiment with your workstation setup and task design to discover what feels best for you. You may find ways to use your old equipment comfortably, or you may need to buy new equipment.

- CHAIR: Your chair should be adjustable. The distance from the floor to the top surface of the seat pan should be equal to the distance from the sole of your shoe to the underside of your thigh. The seat pan should slope slightly forward. It should be fairly flat, with a rounded front edge, and have firm padding. The seat pan should be a length that allows you to lean on the backrest while putting your feet comfortably on the floor. The backrest should be padded and be adjustable to fit into and support the lumbar curve of your back. The chair should probably not have armrests, and if it does, they should not interfere with positioning your arms or the chair itself at the desk.

- DESK: The desk should place your keyboard right where your hands feel best. The desk surface should be at the height that will allow you to sit in the centered position with your hands and arms in their optimal positions for keyboarding. You may need various different surfaces or adjustments to accommodate writing, reading and keyboarding. The desk surface should be wide enough to position the monitor an arm's length away, and your desk should have enough space under it for your legs to be comfortable.

- KEYBOARD: Position your keyboard according to how you use it. If you type primarily on the alphabetic section, then the midpoint of that section should be directly in front of you. The keyboard should be relatively flat rather than slanted. You can level your keyboard by putting adhesive-backed weather stripping tape under the front edge. Ideally, the key action should be light and responsive. You can soften your keys by putting weather stripping squares on them. You will probably be able to use a straight keyboard if you use your hands well, though a V-shaped keyboard may be helpful.

- WRIST SUPPORTS: Wrist supports encourage people to immobilize their hands and put pressure against the underside of their wrists.

- MOUSE: With most keyboards, when you are typing on the alphabetic section and have it centered in front of you, the right end of the keyboard is further from your body's centerline than is the left end. If you put the mouse on your left, it will take less effort to use. Relax your hand on the mouse, and don't push down hard on the button. Don't bend your hand back or let your wrist drag on the desk as you use the mouse. Your mouse button(s) should be light and responsive.

- TRACKBALL: A trackball stays stationary on the desk and takes less effort than a mouse to use. It should be positioned to the left of your keyboard for ordinary alphabetic typing. Keep your wrist straight, and don't rest it on the desk.

- MONITOR: Your monitor should produce clear, sharp images. Dust your screen frequently. Place your monitor directly in front of you at a distance of an arm's length or a bit more. Position the center of the screen so that it is where your gaze naturally falls. Generally, the top of the screen will be about level with your eyes. Tilt the monitor to match the angle of your gaze. Ideally, to rest your eyes, you should position your monitor where you can look out a window or at least across the room.

16

USING LAPTOPS

Computers are wonderful, and laptops are extra wonderful. I write a lot, and after the first time I wrote an article on a computer, I was never able to go back to using a typewriter. When I got my first laptop, I felt free, free to write wherever I was.

I saved this chapter to write on a laptop so that I could live each topic as I wrote it. Most of the chapter I wrote on a trip to Seattle. When I wrote the section on using a laptop at a table, I was using my laptop at a table in the room I was staying in. When I wrote the section on using a laptop sitting on the floor leaning against a wall, I was sitting on the floor in the airport. And of course, I wrote the section about using laptops on an airplane during the flight.

LAPTOP PROBLEMS: However wonderful laptops are for getting work done, they simply cannot be as comfortable as desktop machines. On most laptops, the screen and keyboard are attached and cannot be positioned independently. That means that you cannot simultaneously have both the screen and the keyboard where they should be for comfort. If you position your laptop so that the keyboard is in a fairly comfortable place for typing, then the screen will be much too low and close for comfort. And if you position the top of the screen about eye level, then your laptop's keyboard will be much too high for comfort.

Most laptop users will position the keyboard as well as they can and then lower their heads so they can see the screen, and that will certainly not be a strain-free posture. In addition, the keyboard has to be fairly close to your body for the proper arm position, and this will almost certainly be too close for comfortable use of the eyes. It would be great if laptop screens were detachable and could be positioned for maximum comfort, but that would help only when you had a convenient place to put the screen. As a general rule, you will have to contend with the problem of laptop positioning.

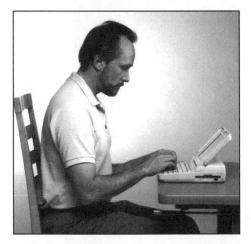

When the table is at standard height, the laptop is too high for comfortable keyboard positioning and too low for comfortable screen positioning. If the table were lower, that would improve the positioning of the arms and make the positioning of the head even worse.

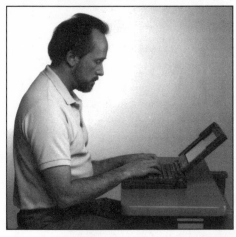

This laptop (a Macintosh Powerbook) has a built in trackball in front of the keys, so the user's hands have to reach to the rear of the laptop to type. When the laptop is too high, the wrists hit the edge of the computer, which can lead to irritation.

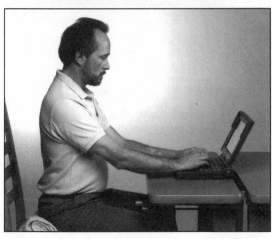

Some users will move the laptop forward to get a better angle of vision. Though this improves the head potion a bit, it is still necessary to look down to use the laptop. Moreover, it puts the hands too far away, which places strain on the shoulders and neck and encourages the user to rest the wrists on the table or the edge of the laptop.

The impossibility of adjusting both the keyboard and monitor for proper comfort suggests that you should not use a laptop as your primary desk computer at your home or office. However, there is a simple, inexpensive solution. You can plug in an external mouse and keyboard and build a stand to put the laptop on. That way you can raise the laptop high enough for proper screen position and still place the keyboard and mouse where they ought to go. Of course, you could also plug an external monitor into your laptop as well and use the laptop simply as a central processing unit. Either of these solutions would make your laptop just as adaptable as a desktop computer.

If you are using your laptop at home or at your office, you can use a desk and chair that will maximize your comfort (see Chapter 15). However, when you are traveling, the problem of finding a tolerable position for laptop use will be complicated by the issues of what you are sitting on and what you are putting your laptop on. If you are traveling, you will have to take what you can get, and what you can get may not be at all what you want.

There is another body use issue that is unique to using laptops. You have to carry the laptop around! You may also have to carry along such extras as an AC adapter, data disks, a set of disks with a backup operating system, an external modem, telephone wire and plugs, extra batteries, a battery charger, a printer and paper, paper documents, and so on. All that is heavy. Carrying the laptop and related equipment is part of using the laptop comfortably, and we will discuss how to avoid discomfort and injuries from carrying your workstation around with you.

What you learned in the first half of this book about comfortable body use applies in using laptops, of course. And even if you don't use a desktop computer at all, you should read the chapter on Desktop Workstations for the information that will apply to laptop use.

The goal in using laptops is to make yourself as comfortable as possible given the limitations of the laptop and the situation in which you are using it. Given the postural constraints of the laptop and the physical strain it can produce, taking time for five-second and three-minute movement breaks will be even more important than with desktop machines.

And when you are traveling with your laptop, don't neglect eating well, getting enough rest and getting some exercise. If you add the stress of neglecting these things to the stress of traveling, you will make yourself much more uncomfortable than you need to be. You can easily do the twenty-minute movement sessions in your hotel room. And one suggestion for those of you who engage in regular exercise at home is to jump rope in your hotel room. It takes no equipment beyond a rope, takes very little space and time, and will give you a good workout.

USING YOUR LAPTOP

Just as with a desktop machine, the first thing to think about in using a laptop is how you sit. That will determine the best level of comfort you can possibly attain. You may have a chair of some kind—an office chair, a couch, a stool, a bench, or whatever. If you are sitting on a chair, you may have your laptop on a support surface, such as a table, a desk, or a chair, or you may have nothing to put it on but your lap. If you have no chair, you may be sitting in bed, on the floor or in some other similar situation. In that case, your laptop may be on your lap or on the floor. Each of these situations has its own requirements for comfort.

When You Have a Chair

In the earlier chapters on sitting and chair use, I recommended using a relatively flat, level chair that can be adjusted for your height. If you have a good chair available, you can use your laptop with the same good posture you learned for sitting at your desktop computer. However, in many situations it will be impossible to get a chair that fits you or that will allow you to sit in the upright, comfortable posture you have learned. In that case, you will have to make do with what you can find.

THE CHAIR: Most chairs have a seat pan and backrest that slant back. In addition, most chairs have a seat pan that has some degree of bucket, and many chairs have a backrest that is concave to some degree. A fat, cushy easy chair or a soft couch are the extreme of this concave, non-supportive chair design. Sitting in a chair that is to one degree or another non-supportive forces you into a slumped posture. Your pelvis will roll back, your back will round, and your chest will cave in.

Such a chair does not offer the support that allows proper pelvic positioning, so you will wind up leaning against the backrest. The best you can do in most cases is to put something behind you—a pillow, a sweater, and so on—to fill in the concavity in the backrest. In this case, I actually do recommend using a lumbar support. You will find that it will considerably reduce the strain of sitting in a bad chair. You may also find that putting something like a towel, a blanket, or even a telephone book under you can help. If the chair has a bucket, you can fill in some of the bucket that way. If the chair is too soft, that will make the seat pan harder and flatter. And if the chair is too low, sitting on something will raise you up. If you are forced to use a less than comfortable chair, pay attention to keeping your posture as open as possible, and take frequent rest and movement breaks.

THE TABLE: When you are positioning your laptop on a desk or table, it is really the keyboard that you are positioning, and that is essentially the same as positioning your desktop computer keyboard on a desk or table. A key consideration is the height of the table. Just as with an ordinary desktop keyboard, positioning the laptop too high will result in a lot of strain on your arms, hands, shoulders, neck, and back. If you are traveling and are using your laptop at a desk or table that is not yours, you will probably not be able to adjust the height to your exact needs. If the desk you are sitting at is too high, often the best you will be able to do by way of adjustment is to sit on a pillow or telephone book. If the desk is too low, put your laptop on top of a book, a folded blanket or whatever you can find.

THE SCREEN: Once you have found a way to sit as comfortably as possible in the chair you have available and have adjusted the table height as well as you can, you will still have to deal with the position of the screen. The screen will be too low and will probably be too close for comfort, and there's not much you can do about that.

Be sure to experiment with the tilt of the screen. You will have to line the screen up as well as possible with your line of sight. To some extent, tilting the screen away from you can increase its distance, but if you go too far, the display will lose its sharpness and be hard to read. You will also want to adjust screen tilt to reduce glare from light sources.

You will have to look down at the screen for some or all of your work time, and that will be fatiguing. There are two partial solutions.

If you look again at the picture of my son reading (in Chapter 4), you will see that even with the book on the floor, he maintains his erect posture. To look down, he rotates his head rather than collapsing his torso. If you lengthen your back and rotate your head down, as my son does in the picture, that will help somewhat in looking at your laptop screen. To rotate your head, sit erect and raise the back of your head slightly while moving your face down. However, even this position may not be comfortable for most people for long periods of time.

Another partial solution is to sit upright and look straight out into the room as you type, looking at the screen as little as possible. You will still have to look down occasionally to make sure of what is on the screen, but looking straight out will help—if you can touch type and if your work is primarily text entry that doesn't demand constant attention to the screen.

ON YOUR LAP: In many situations, you will be using your laptop without any desk at all. Sitting with the laptop on your lap makes the problem of looking down at the screen even worse, but some partial solutions are available.

You may find yourself sitting upright in a good chair, or you may find yourself sitting in more or less of a reclining position in a less supportive chair. In either case, there are two basic ways that you can sit on a chair with a laptop on your lap. You may sit with your knees together and the laptop balanced on your knees, or you may sit with one ankle crossed over your other knee.

Sitting with your laptop balanced on both your knees is fairly comfortable. Laptop keyboards generally don't have number pads, so you can balance the whole keyboard centered on your knees. It is true that your knees must be close together. Ordinarily I do not recommend this position since it creates some tension in your back and breathing, but having both feet flat on floor does provide fair stability and balance for supporting your laptop.

Sitting with one foot crossed over the other knee, however, is problematic. Sitting this way repositions the hip of the leg that is up. It tilts your pelvis back and rounds your lower back, and it tips your pelvis to one side and curves your spinal column sideways. In addition, having one foot off the floor makes the posture as a whole less balanced and stable. The compression and imbalance created by this posture will result in strain on your neck and arms if you sit this way for long.

However, since you are sitting on whatever you can find, and it probably isn't very comfortable anyway, moving from one less-than-comfortable position to another will offer a change of posture and support, and for this reason you may find yourself dropping into the crossed-leg position now and again. When you do, pay attention to keeping your posture as open and lengthened as possible rather than allowing the unbalanced posture to force you into collapsing your body.

Pay attention to how you hold your arms and shoulders when your laptop is on your lap. If you lean back in the chair and adopt a reclining sitting posture, your laptop will be fairly far in front of you on your lap and you will have to reach your hands out too far forward to get to the keys. That will drag your shoulders forward, down and together, which will fatigue and strain not only your shoulders but your neck and back.

As much as possible, sit upright with the laptop pulled toward you so your arms don't have to reach too far forward. Make sure that you let your shoulders relax. Don't hold your hands in position by hiking up your shoulders, and make sure to rest your arms by moving them around frequently rather than staying in a position of static holding. Also, make sure to stop typing and put your arms down for a rest now and again.

With No Chair

There may be times when you use your laptop with no chair at all. You may be sitting in bed in your hotel room late at night working. You may be out in the woods writing poetry. Or you may be sitting on the floor in an airport, either because all the seats are taken or because you want to get close enough to a socket to plug your laptop in. How you sit when you have no chair to sit on depends first on whether you have a backrest or not. It also depends on whether you sit with your legs crossed or straight out in front of you.

I started this book on the floor. I usually begin complex writing projects by typing into a file random ideas as they occur to me over the course of months of reading and preparation. Then I print out the file, cut the sheets of paper into strips with one idea per strip, and physically arrange the strips into an outline. At one point in writing this book I had a couple of hundred idea slips all arranged on my living room floor. I brought my laptop in, sat in the middle of it all like a spider in a web of ideas, and began writing the book. I don't normally sit on the floor to use a computer, but I did then.

WITH A BACKREST: We'll start by assuming you are sitting on the floor or ground in a cross-legged position. If you have a backrest such as a wall or a tree, that may offer the most comfortable way of sitting, but you would need a pillow or rolled up blanket to use as a lumbar support. Without that support, leaning back onto a flat surface would result in severe and uncomfortable rounding of your back and collapsing of your chest.

Once you are sitting, you also have to place your laptop on something. If you put it on the floor in front of you, you will have to lean forward away from the backrest or slump to get your shoulders far enough forward and down for your hands to reach the keyboard. Putting your laptop on your lap will be most comfortable. It is best to use a rolled up jacket or blanket or something of the sort under the laptop when it is on your lap—if you have anything with you that you can use. That raises it up a bit to a spot that your hands can reach more comfortably, and it provides a soft surface on which it will be easier to get your laptop level.

The alternative to using a back support is to use a rolled towel for pelvic support as we did on a chair, but in this instance trying to use the upright posture will probably result in a lot of discomfort. If you keep your pelvis and back aligned to an upright position and sit up tall, then the screen of your laptop will be very far down on your lap. In order to see it at all, you will have to rotate your head quite far down, which will strain your neck.

On the whole, I think leaning back against a back support and using a lumbar support is a better position if you do have to type on the floor with your laptop on your lap. Of course, your head will be held somewhat forward, which ordinarily is not a good idea. Make sure to take rest breaks and movement breaks frequently.

You may find it helpful to experiment with having the laptop slant slightly away from you. If you have your laptop down on your lap, you may have to hold your hands lower than would be comfortable and bend your hands backward at the wrist a bit to get them flat for typing. Slanting the keyboard away from you may allow your wrists to straighten out a bit.

WITHOUT A BACKREST: If you are sitting without a backrest and simply put your laptop on the floor, you will find it very fatiguing. You will have to lean forward quite a bit to type on it. Your arms will be too far out in front of you, and it will be fatiguing to hold them there. If you sit upright, your hands will have to be bent severely back to type on the keyboard. If you slump down, that repositions your arms so they are farther forward and your hands are flatter, but your back will be rounded, and your head will be far forward with no support. I am sitting this way now as I type, and it is very uncomfortable. Don't sit this way if you have any choice at all.

There are two ways to sit on the floor with no back support and use your laptop comfortably. Sit in the centered posture, with a towel roll for pelvic support. If you have a box or another rolled up blanket or something of the sort, you can put it on the floor in front of you and put your laptop down on it. That moves your laptop a bit farther forward and raises it up a bit, which reduces the bend in your neck required to see the screen and improves the hand position on the keyboard. To sit this way, you must be flexible enough to cross your legs and get your knees flat on the floor. This can actually be quite comfortable, though not as comfortable as typing on a desktop computer.

A variation on this way of sitting is to sit on top of some firm cushions or folded blankets, with your feet on the floor. This lowers your legs and helps arch your back, which relieves some of the strain of sitting with no backrest. (See the Knee–Hips Height experiment in Chapter 8.) You would need a higher box or even a low chair to put your laptop on.

LEG POSITION: In the discussion so far, we have assumed you had no chair and were sitting with your legs crossed. Most people cross their ankles when they sit cross-legged on the floor. They put each knee on top of the inside edge of the opposite foot. However, in this posture, one knee is raised slightly higher, which tips your pelvis to one side and imbalances your sitting posture. Though it is only a slight tip, it does reduce your stability a bit and increases the effort needed to maintain a sitting position. If you sit this way, make sure to periodically switch which leg is in front.

The best position for sitting cross-legged on the floor actually has your legs *folded* rather than crossed. Both your knees and ankles are on the floor, and you can maintain a balanced sitting position. (If you look again at the picture of my son, you will see that is how he is sitting.) Of course, many people are not flexible enough to rest their knees on the floor, and that presents a problem. The stretching exercises described in Chapter 13 will do a lot to help you increase your flexibility enough to sit this way.

Sitting with your knees up in the air will round your low back and collapse your posture. If your knees are up, it will be very difficult to sit upright using pelvic support and no backrest. If you are sitting against a back support, raising your knees will still round your back and collapse your neck, but it won't be as much of a problem. You will be leaning back onto the back support and you won't have to hold your own body weight up. This is still a collapsed posture, so it will be important to take frequent movement and rest breaks.

However, aside from the strain on your neck and arms, sitting cross-legged with your knees up will also put strain on your legs. The reason that your knees won't go down to the floor is that certain ligaments and muscles around your hips are too short to allow that movement. The weight of your legs dragging down on those ligaments and muscles will create strain. Adding the weight of your laptop could be very uncomfortable. In order to support your legs and take the strain off, you could put a pillow under each knee.

A very different option would be to lean back against a support and put your legs out straight in front of you. That is probably a better position if you do not have the flexibility to sit with your legs folded. It rounds the back, but using a towel for pelvic support, along with something for lumbar support behind your back, will help. Again, your neck will be somewhat collapsed, and frequent breaks will be important.

STRADDLE SITTING: There is one other position I'd like to mention, and that is using a laptop straddling a bench. By that I mean sitting with one leg on either side of the bench, as though you were sitting on a horse. If you put the laptop on the bench in front of you, that sitting posture will be very similar to sitting on the floor with no back support and with the laptop on the floor in front of you. Here too you should use a pelvic support and put the laptop on something to raise it up.

Though there are many other situations and positions in which you could use your laptop, I will leave it to you to figure out how, based on your knowledge of the principles of proper posture and body use. The positions covered here ought to be enough for most people.

On an Airplane

Using laptops on airplanes deserves a section of its own. People often use laptops on airplanes, and airplane seats are particularly difficult. For whatever reason, they have been designed to approximate sitting inside a padded sphere. The seats are actually concave, and they lead to a grossly slumped posture. They force your pelvis to roll back and your chest to collapse. As I type this, I am sitting exactly that way in a seat on my flight to Seattle. I can feel my neck collapsing and straining and my arms beginning to tense up.

The first thing I do whenever I board an airplane is get two pillows to fill in the hollow in the backrest. That actually makes the airplane seat almost comfortable. As I type this, I have put two small pillows behind my back, and I am much less compressed and much more comfortable. If you cannot get pillows, a blanket, coat or anything of the sort will do.

A particular feature of airplane seating is the rather narrow seat with armrests on both sides. I am thin and not very tall, yet I find the seat to be narrow and confining. When there are people sitting on either side of me, I cannot pull up the armrests and spread out. The seat is so narrow that I cannot even comfortably position my elbows inside the armrests but am almost forced to place my arms up on the armrests, which puts me in a bind. If I rest my arms on the arm rests, that irritates my elbows and forearms a bit. If I hold them up to lessen the weight, that fatigues my shoulders. And if I hold them tight to my body to get them positioned inside the armrests, that also makes my shoulders and neck tense. I find that I prefer holding my elbows inside the armrests. If you find putting your arms on the armrests more comfortable, you might think about putting a pad of some sort on the armrests to cushion them and protect your arms. Of course, if there is no one on either side of you, raise the armrests and let your arms fall down into their position of natural comfort.

Sitting on an airplane, there is so little leg room that it is generally not comfortable to cross one ankle over your other knee. That means that you have two choices for laptop support. You can keep your feet on the floor and put the computer on your lap, or you can put your laptop on the fold-down tray table located on the back of the seat in front of you. If you put the laptop on your lap, the keyboard is lower and so, of course, is the screen.

If you choose to put your computer on the tray table, the keyboard is considerably higher up. Some tray tables slide forward and back, and others don't, which affects the placement of the keyboard. Again, you want to place the keyboard close enough to you that you don't fatigue your arms by holding them too far away from your body. Depending on your height, you may or may not find that having the keyboard higher up will be comfortable. Make sure that having the keyboard up doesn't force you to raise your hands so high that your shoulders and arms become uncomfortable. In particular, make sure that you don't rest your wrists against the edge of the computer or the tray table. That could result in considerable discomfort. Another element to consider is that having the screen up higher will reduce how much you need to bend your head forward to see the screen. That can be a major factor in your comfort.

Laptops with Trackballs

Most computers now employ a Graphical User Interface, which depends on the use of a mouse to control many screen elements. Many laptop computers have built-in trackballs, since it would be inconvenient or impossible to use a mouse while traveling. Some laptop computers have a trackpad instead of a trackball, but the placement and use of the trackpad is essentially the same as for the trackball.

On laptops with no trackballs, the keys are located on the edge of the laptop closest to the user. On the laptops with trackballs, the trackball is placed on a flat "shelf" that occupies the half of the laptop surface closest to the user, and the keys occupy the half farther away, right below the screen. Since many people will be coping with the positioning effects of this keyboard design, it is worth devoting a bit of space to how to use this configuration comfortably.

The first consideration in using a laptop with a trackball is to make sure that the computer is positioned close enough to you that you don't have to reach your hands out too far forward to get to the keys.

You will have to position the laptop closer to you than a laptop with no trackball simply to get the keys close enough for comfort.

You may be tempted to position the laptop farther from you and ease the strain on your arms by resting your wrists on the flat surface beside the trackball, but that would be similar to using a wrist rest on a desktop computer. (See the earlier photographs illustrating the postural difficulties associated with laptop use.) Resting your wrists near the trackball will put pressure on your wrists and could lead to irritation there. Pay attention to how your wrists feel. If you do rest your wrists on the trackball surface, make sure to lift your hands if there is the slightest hint of discomfort from pressure on your wrists. However, don't lift your wrists by hiking up your shoulders. Pay attention to letting your shoulders relax. Make sure to move your arms frequently rather than staying in a position of static holding, and make sure to put your arms down for a rest now and again.

If you are using your trackball-equipped laptop on a table or desk, the height is even more important than for other laptops. If the table is too high, you will find that reaching past the trackball surface will be very difficult, and you may well find that the edge of the computer closest to you will press into your wrists. In that case, find a lower surface for the laptop or put pillows on your chair to raise yourself up higher. You could also put a book or other support under the rear edge of the laptop. By tilting the whole keyboard toward you, you make it easier to get your hands past the front edge. If worst comes to worst, you could simply put the laptop on your lap.

Using a trackball-equipped laptop on an airplane presents a special problem. Putting the computer on the tray table may raise it so high that the front edge cuts into your wrists as you reach forward to get to the keys. When I used a laptop with a trackball on a flight, that was exactly the situation I ran into, and I found that the only way I could use it comfortably was by putting it on my lap.

CARRYING YOUR LAPTOP

Lifting and carrying your laptop are part of using it, and you may experience fatigue and strain, or even injuries, from improper body use. Proper lifting and carrying are important. In just a moment, we will do some exercises on proper lifting and carrying, but first let's look at four rules for good body use in these tasks.

BASIC RULES: First, *keep your computer and accessories as close to your body as possible when lifting or carrying.* The farther away from your body you position your load, the greater the leverage it exerts on your body and the greater the strain. When you lift your laptop carrying case, place yourself close to it and lift as much straight upward as possible. Don't stand far away, lean over, and hoist it up toward you. When you carry your laptop, hold it close to your body.

Second, *lift with a straight, upward movement.* Do not bend forward or sideways and lift with an arcing movement. It is especially important not to use a twisting movement to lift something from beside you and bring the load around in front of you. Lifting with a twisting motion places a great deal of strain on your back and can easily lead to injuries.

Third, *use your legs for lifting.* The way to keep the load close to you and use straight upward movements is to keep the weight joined to the vertical center line of your body. Use the muscles of your legs rather than the muscles of your back and arms to lift.

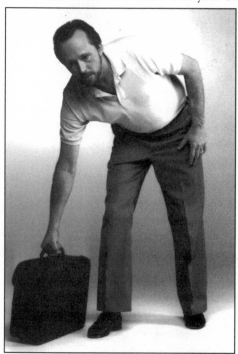

The wrong way to lift a laptop—bending, twisting and reaching puts a dangerous strain on the back.

Fourth, *maintain a lengthened, opened body use while lifting and carrying.* Let your body gently lengthen upward rather than collapsing to support the weight of your laptop. (See the discussion in Chapter 13 on lengthened body use.)

CARRYING CASES: Before we consider just how to lift and carry a laptop, it will be important to think about what you will carry it in, since that will determine how you lift and carry your laptop. Most people carry their laptops in shoulder bags or briefcases, and many briefcases have shoulder straps as well as handles. Whether you use a shoulder bag or a briefcase, the weight of your laptop will rest on one side of your body, and this can present a problem.

Watch someone walking along carrying a suitcase in one hand or with a bag slung over one shoulder. How do they compensate for the weight being carried on one side of their body? They lean sideways and down to the opposite side. This illustrates a basic fact of body use. In order to support weight held on one side, some body part has to move out to the other side to balance it. However, when people bend sideways and down, they usually collapse and compress the side of their body that they lean toward. This creates fatigue and strain. Even worse, most people have a preferred side. They most frequently carry weights on that side of their body,

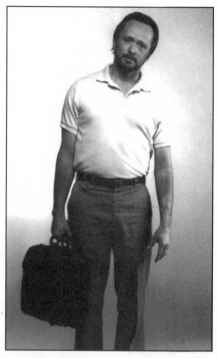

Leaning to the left will compress the left side and will be not be comfortable.

thereby concentrating the strain on just one side. (For an example of better body use, see the photographs in the upcoming experiment on Lifting Your Shoulder Bag or Knapsack.)

If you use a shoulder bag or briefcase, the weight will hang on your shoulder, which will fatigue your shoulder and neck. If you use a briefcase, you will also experience a good deal of strain in your forearms, wrists, and hands from supporting the weight of your laptop on your curled fingers. If you have any wrist strain from typing, extra wrist strain from holding your briefcase is the last thing you need.

The thickness of the shoulder bag or briefcase is also important. The thicker it is, the harder it will be to hold close to your side. If the carrying case is thick, weight will be carried farther from your side, which will increase the length of the lever arm and make it harder to carry the briefcase. It will be easier to hold a shoulder bag or briefcase if it stores your materials in a longer, thinner shape.

There are clearly difficulties with using a shoulder bag or briefcase. Instead, you might consider carrying your laptop in a knapsack. Yes, I know a knapsack wouldn't present the proper business image, but before we talk about that, let's consider the advantages it has to offer. With a knapsack, the weight is held close to your body and positioned along the center of your body rather than along one side. That way the bones and muscles of the core of the body can do a better job of supporting the weight of the laptop. You don't have to bend sideways to counterbalance the weight of the laptop. You may bend forward a bit, but that is a much less imbalanced and strained position to hold.

Security may be also important to you. I don't know how often laptops are the objects of attention for thieves, but depending on your equipment, you could be carrying around five or six thousand dollars in a small package. A knapsack will not be so obviously identifiable as containing a laptop computer, and it will be much harder to tear away from you than a shoulder bag or a briefcase.

You can buy knapsacks that are designed for carrying laptops. You can also buy roomy multi-compartmented general purpose knapsacks that work wonderfully for carrying a laptop. If the knapsack has a padded hip strap, that is a definite plus. The hip strap belt enables you to load the weight of the knapsack onto your hips. This is far more comfortable than supporting the weight on your shoulders if you will be carrying the knapsack for any distance. If you are going to be carrying a heavy knapsack a long distance, it will also help to use a bandanna to tie the shoulder straps together at chest height. Or you could buy a sternum strap at an outdoor store. That will take more of the weight of the knapsack off your shoulders and allow your chest to support some of it.

A little tip. If you are using a general purpose knapsack, it will not include the padding necessary for protecting a laptop from the inevitable jolts that traveling will bring. Go to a camping supply store and buy one of the cheaper foam rubber ground covers campers put under their sleeping bags. In just a few minutes, with some duct tape, you can create a foam box that you can insert into your knapsack to protect your computer.

Now to the fact that knapsacks don't have the right image for trim, well-dressed business people. To begin with, ask yourself which is more important, your business image or the safety of your back. You may have to make a choice in favor of your back. On the other hand, I do realize that people's expected images do form part of the operating environment for someone in business, and though a knapsack is comfortable, there may be situations in which you will not be able to use one. However, you can buy a convertible briefcase/knapsack designed specifically for laptops. This kind of carrying case has shoulder straps that can be tucked into a compartment and hidden.

You can use it as a knapsack when you need to carry it for long periods and as a briefcase when you need to look like a business person. There are other general purpose convertible knapsacks that include hip belts as well as shoulder straps, both of which can be zipped into hidden compartments.

If you feel you cannot use a knapsack, the next best solution will be to use a carrying case that has both a shoulder strap and a hand grip. Switching from one to the other may help. It will also be very important to switch the case from side to side periodically in order to share the weight between your two sides. And you could get a small luggage carrier with wheels to put your laptop and other luggage on so that you can avoid carrying your laptop as much as possible.

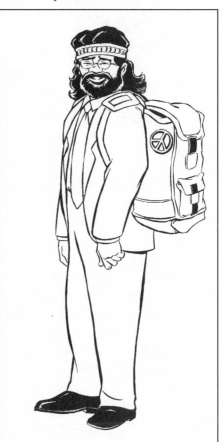

Are you afraid that using a backpack will present the wrong image? It is worth it to save your back.

LIFTING YOUR LAPTOP: Now let's look at the best ways of lifting your laptop in its case.

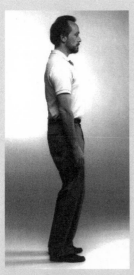

EXPERIMENT: BENDING YOUR KNEES

Stand up and bend your knees. When you bend your knees, do you lean forward or keep your back vertical? Do you tuck your tail or arch your back? How far down can you go while keeping your feet flat on the floor?

Many people keep their torsos pretty much vertical and tuck their tails when they bend their knees, but this restricts the movement and reduces overall balance. Try the movement again, but this time as you bend your knees, lean your chest forward a bit and stick your tailbone out backward a bit. You may need to arch your back slightly to stick your tail out, but make sure it is a gentle, relaxed movement

Tucking the tail and keeping the back vertical limits the movement of bending.

rather than a tense, effortful one. This pelvic movement is the opposite of tucking your tail. Bending your knees while rotating your pelvis forward puts the focus of the movement on your legs rather than your low back. (This is related to the Airport Duck experiment in Chapter 8.) It leads to freer, stronger movement of your legs and better balance on your feet, which will be important in lifting your laptop.

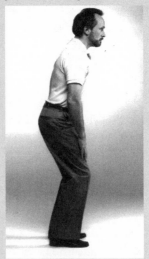

Bending from the legs/hips allows a freer and stronger movement.

Some people may feel uncomfortable about sticking their tail out, but it is a natural and important movement, nothing that people should worry about. This "squatting" position is the ready or power position in a wide variety of sports and movement activities. It is a basic element in safe, strong body use.

EXPERIMENT: LIFTING YOUR LAPTOP

Stand upright with your laptop briefcase on the floor beside your feet. You may wish to start practicing with a very light load in your briefcase rather than your full travel load.

As you have undoubtedly heard many times, you have to lift with your legs, not your back. To get into position to do that, bend your knees, and at the same time stick your tail out behind you. This will result in a "squatting" position, with your knees bent, your torso leaning somewhat forward, and your back in its normal, straight (but not vertical) alignment. That will help you squat down from your hips and avoid rounding your back. Keeping your back straight rather than bending it will vastly reduce the strain of lifting. In this crouched position, grasp the handle of your briefcase.

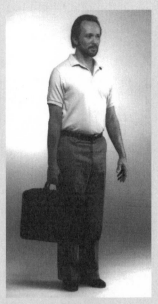

Notice the lengthened, balanced, upright carrying posture.

Now, lift your laptop by straightening your knees and rising to standing. If you extend the arm that is not grasping the carrying case out to the side, that provides a lateral counterbalance to the weight of the case and makes the lifting easier. (If you aren't altogether sure why I recommend not tucking your tail when you lift, bend your knees, tuck your tail, grasp the handle of your briefcase, and lift your laptop this way. Be careful. It can put a strain on your back.)

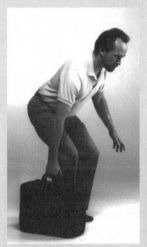
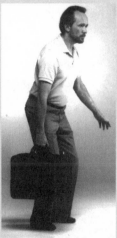

Lifting with a straight up movement—by using the legs, not the back.

If you are using a briefcase, then this lifting motion is all you need. If you are using a shoulder bag or a knapsack, then your movement will be a bit different since you have to get a shoulder strap or two into place. In lifting a shoulder bag or knapsack, it is very important to avoid a twisting/lifting movement, which could injure your back.

EXPERIMENT:
LIFTING YOUR SHOULDER BAG OR KNAPSACK

Stand with your shoulder bag on the floor in front of your feet. Hold the shoulder strap with both hands. Assuming you are right handed and want to use your right hand for primary support and manipulation, hold the strap with your right hand near the middle of its length. Put your right hand under the strap and your left hand over the strap, with a bit of space between your hands. Bend your knees and then straighten your legs to lift the shoulder bag up in front of you.

That movement gives you a straight up lift. How will you get it around onto your shoulder? Don't swing the bag around you, which would require a twist of your torso. Instead, move your body into position under the bag. The key is to keep your body vertical and spin your whole body on its vertical axis.

There is a fairly simple way to do this. After you have lifted the shoulder bag and have it up around shoulder height, spin your body to the left by taking a short step forward with your right foot. Simultaneously lift the shoulder bag up higher with your right hand. That movement leaves the shoulder bag almost where it was in midair and spins your body into position under it, which avoids side-bending or twisting your body. In order to put the shoulder bag down safely, just reverse the order of these movements.

There is a second way to get the shoulder bag onto your shoulder. It is a more economical movement, but some people may find the coordination more difficult. From the same initial position, lift straight up and simultaneously take a step back with your right foot. Make sure to keep your body erect and untwisted. That will spin your body around in a clockwise movement as you lift, and it will pull the shoulder bag into a rising, spiraling movement. Rather than making the lift two distinct movements with two distinct directions, you will be lifting the shoulder bag in one smooth spiral of movement. If you can do it without bending sideways or twisting at your waist, you will find it a smoother, easier movement.

Two ways of lifting a shoulder bag or knapsack

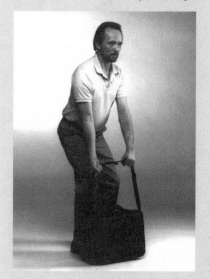
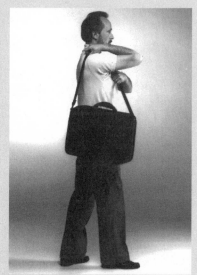

The easier way to lift a laptop is to step forward with the right foot and turn into position under the laptop.

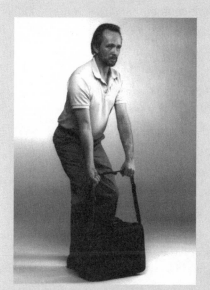
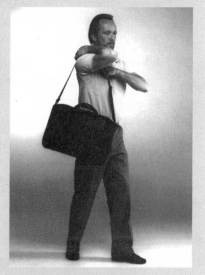

The more economical way to lift a laptop is to step backward with the right foot while lifting and swinging the laptop up into position, all in one movement.

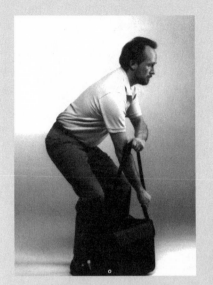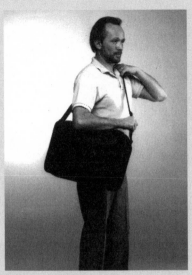

Hand position for placing the strap across the shoulders.

Lifting a knapsack uses exactly the same movements. The only difference is that you have two shoulder straps to work with. Hold the right shoulder strap and follow all the directions as though you were lifting a shoulder bag. At the end, after you have gotten the right strap on your right shoulder, you can easily slip your left arm through the left shoulder strap if you have loosened it enough before lifting your knapsack.

There is one more consideration about lifting a shoulder bag. I have been describing a movement in which the shoulder strap is placed on the shoulder on the same side as you carry your bag on. You might want to place the shoulder strap across your body on the shoulder on the opposite side. How do you get the shoulder strap across your back without awkward, dangerous bending/twisting/lifting movements? This may be harder or easier depending on the weight of your bag and the length of the shoulder strap. If you have to lift your laptop and put it down frequently, you may find that crossing and uncrossing the strap over your body is too much work.

If you have back problems, the safest way would be to lift the shoulder bag up, rest it on a table, and then simply put the shoulder strap across your body. Of course, if you have back problems, you probably shouldn't carry a shoulder bag. Another way to do the lift is very similar to the lift you have already done. The difference is in how your hold your hands. Assuming you will lift the bag up to your right side, stand as you did initially. But this time cross your hands. Put your left hand, palm down, around the middle of the strap. Put your right hand, palm down, near the left end of the strap. Do the initial lift as you did before. But when it comes time to put the strap over your head, support most of the weight of the bag with your right hand. That will free your left hand to move the strap over your head and across your shoulders. Make sure not to bend or twist your neck and back as you move the strap.

CARRYING YOUR LAPTOP: Once you have the laptop up, you will have to pay attention to lengthened carrying. The lengthened body line I showed in the section on movement breaks (Chapter 13) is even more important in carrying your laptop case. Since your body is carrying weight, postural mistakes can lead to significant strain and pain. If you let your body collapse and compress, you will strain your back and fatigue your whole body. It is possible to use your body in a lengthened, opened line rather than a collapsed, compressed bend, and you will find that this will be much more comfortable.

There is one other carrying situation you are likely to face, and that is carrying both your laptop and a suitcase. If you carry your laptop in a briefcase, you could carry it on one side and the suitcase on the other. You would lift the laptop as described earlier, but with a weight in each hand. Having a weight in each hand will result in better balancing of the whole body. The laptop will probably be in a smaller case, so you should bend your knees and lift that case first. Then bend your knees and lift the suitcase next. If you are using a shoulder case, lift it first and then the suitcase.

EXPERIMENT: LENGTHENED CARRYING

When you carry your laptop in a briefcase or shoulder case, you will tend to lean to the side away from the case to counterbalance the weight of the case. If you are carrying the case on your right, you will lean to the left. However, rather than leaning leftward by shortening and compressing your left side, lengthen your torso. Reach up and out to the left with the right side of your body. That doesn't mean to hike up your right shoulder. Make sure your right shoulder is relaxed and down. Opening your right side means standing with good support on your left leg and reaching in an upward and leftward arc with your whole right side, from your sole to your neck and head. (See the photographs in the experiment on Lifting Your Shoulder Bag or Knapsack.)

Lengthened carrying applies with knapsacks as well. If your knapsack is heavy, you will notice a tendency to counterbalance it by leaning your body forward. Rather than bending forward by collapsing your chest, lean forward by lengthening forward and up along the whole back side of your body. That lengthens your body and frees it.

Even though having a suitcase in one hand and a laptop in the other is a nicely balanced situation, I find it more comfortable to use a suitcase along with a knapsack. Using a briefcase, I have to maintain a constant grip on a handle with each hand, but with a knapsack, I can shift the suitcase back and forth and rest one hand. Using a shoulder case, would free up one hand but I find it very fatiguing on my neck and shoulder. Of course, using a suitcase with wheels makes the best sense because then you don't have to pick up and carry that weight.

These are some thoughts about how to use a laptop. If you pay attention to the ways you use and carry your laptop, you will find that you can be a comfortable computer user and a strong packhorse as well.

KEY POINTS

- Laptops cannot be as comfortable as desktop machines since the screen and keyboard generally cannot be positioned independently. The screen will usually be too close and too low for optimal body use. *However, plugging in an external keyboard and mouse and putting the laptop up on a stand allow proper, comfortable use of the laptop.*

- When you travel, you may not have an appropriate chair or desk to use. Pay attention to your body use. Sit as well as you can, and take frequent movement and rest breaks. Experiment with different ways to sit and position your laptop.

- When you work on an airplane, make sure to fill in the concave backrest with a pillow or two.

- If your laptop has a trackball shelf in front of the keyboard, make sure not to let it press into your wrists as you type.

- Lifting and carrying your laptop wrong can lead to pain and injuries. To decrease the strain, keep your laptop as close to your body as possible when lifting or carrying. Lift by using a straight upward movement that comes from your legs. Be very careful not to lift by bending and twisting your back. Lengthen your body to carry your laptop safely and comfortably.

- To carry your laptop in the most balanced and strain-free way, use a knapsack.

17

STANDING WORKSTATION

$\mathbf{S}$tanding workstations are often used to allow people enough
mobility to do many related tasks. Airline ticket agents, for example, must enter passenger information into a computer, move pas-
sengers' suitcases onto the scales, and then move the suitcases to
conveyor belts. Nurses frequently have standing computer workstations, as do librarians and sales clerks.

Very often, people working at a standing workstation have to hand
write information onto paper documents as well as key information
into a computer. Their workstation, therefore, must allow them to
perform both movement tasks comfortably.

The fundamental rules of proper body use and workstation setup
still apply to standing computer use. The basic elements to consider
are posture and relaxation, keyboard placement and monitor placement. An additional factor may be multi-person use of the workstation. If many people use your workstation, any adjustments you
make will have to be easy to do and undo.

STANDING POSTURE
In order to figure out the best keyboard and monitor placement, you
must start by considering how to balance your body as you stand.
Sitting involves balancing the torso, head, and arms on the pelvis.
Standing adds the additional factor of balancing the pelvis (and
everything above it) on top of the legs. Imagine a column of blocks.
The more blocks in the column, and the higher the column, the
harder it is to balance. Bringing the extra joints of the knees, ankles,
and feet into the process of postural balance makes balancing the
body in a standing position even more complex than balancing it
when sitting.

Think back to the chapter on Improving Use of Your legs (Chapter 8). Remember the sense of vitality you achieved with the proper organization of your walking. That same energized posture is the key to working comfortably at a standing computer workstation. Your body has to be balanced over its centerline. It has to be erect and lengthened upwards, and your weight has to be balanced comfortably on your feet.

You have to hold your arms out front to type. Some sales workstations utilize a touch-sensitive computer screen, which also requires that one or both hands be held out forward. Holding your arms out forward can cause fatigue or back strain, as can raising and lowering your arms frequently. Let's examine how your arms can best be supported by your body in a standing position. The key is that your feet, legs, and pelvis must be directly involved in the weight shifts that are part of raising your arms, holding them up, and lowering them.

EXPERIMENT: ARMS AND STANDING BALANCE

Stand up with your arms down by your sides. Now lift your arms forward and up, to shoulder height in front of you. Try this movement a few times. As you lift your arms up, what adjustments do you make with your body? Do you move your shoulders or your pelvis? Does the weight shift on your feet? If you wish to amplify the effects of this experiment, hold a telephone book or something of the sort with both your hands as you raise your arms. (If you have back or neck problems, you may find lifting any weight out in front of you at arm's length to be a significant strain. Be careful not to further injure yourself. It may be safer for you not to try lifting anything.)

Did you move your shoulders back as you lifted your arms forward? Most people do. Moving your shoulders back serves to counterbalance the weight of your arms extending out in front of your body. However, moving your shoulders back arches your back, making you lean back and put extra weight and pressure on your low back. If you hold this posture for any length of time, you will probably feel strain in the back of your neck and in your low back.

With your arms down by your sides, lengthen your posture upward. Let your belly relax. Let your breath fall down into your belly and your weight fall down into your feet. Now as you raise your arms, bend your knees very slightly and move your tailbone ever so slightly to your rear. Don't arch your back to move your tailbone, but instead move your whole pelvis rearward a slight bit. You may wish to tuck your tail a slight bit as you do this, if you need to prevent yourself from arching your back. But don't go into a fully tucked position. Make sure your knees are not locked. Moving the weight of your pelvis to the rear will counterbalance the weight of your arms moving forward and up. That will help you avoid arching and straining your back.

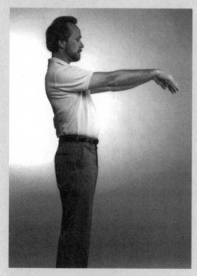 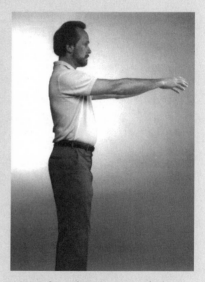

Using the shoulders to counter-balance the arm movement strains the back.

Using the pelvis to counterbalance the arm movements creates a stronger, freer posture.

Actually, many people walk around all the time with their shoulders back, their backs arched, and the weight of their upper bodies hanging on their low backs. It is a common source of back strain. If this is the normal posture you bring to working at a standing workstation, you may be adding injury to insult. It will be very important to open and lengthen your standing posture.

EXPERIMENT: STANDING POSTURE

Stand and feel your posture. If you wish to see your posture, you could have someone videotape you, or you could simply stand in front of a video camera and watch yourself on the TV. A low tech option is to go to a clothing store and stand in front of the three-panel mirror used for trying on clothes.

Do you stand in the slumped arch just described? If you do, there is a way to change that. Feel your heels on the floor. Imagine/feel a line of movement starting at your heels, lifting upward along the backs of your legs, and lifting upward along your back. When it gets to about shoulder blade level, arc the line smoothly forward and up to a point somewhere above and in front of your head. Make sure that in imaging the line you don't lift your shoulders or try to pull yourself up. The process will be gentle and subtle when you do it right.

As your body gently follows the line forward and up, you will rise out of the slump and attain a lighter, more architecturally balanced standing posture. You will find that this posture will make the Feet Walking exercise (in Chapter 8) easier and more effective.

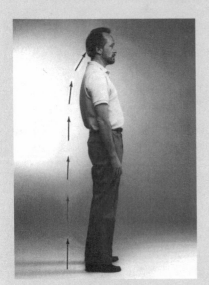 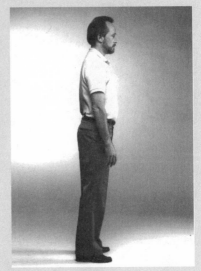

Moving up and out of a collapsed standing posture

Needless to say, there are many many different ways to unbalance the human body. If you feel that you would benefit from postural work, you can find a body awareness educator or other knowledgeable professional who could analyze your particular ways of using your body.

One brief comment should be made about a common recommendation for standing posture. Often the advice is given to stand with one foot on a low stool and tuck your tail if you will be standing for lengthy periods. This is said to take the strain off the low back. However, if you try it, you will find that it will tend to tip your pelvis to the side, which actually increases imbalance and strain in your hips, back and legs.

By using your pelvis as the core of your posture, you can maintain a balanced and erect standing position in front of your computer keyboard. If you maintain this erect standing posture, you will find that you use your torso, head and arms in the same way both sitting and standing. Your head and torso will be vertical, balanced and free.

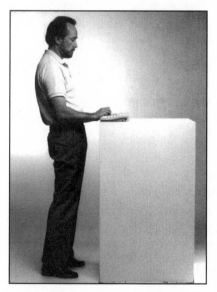

Using a keyboard with a collapsed standing posture.

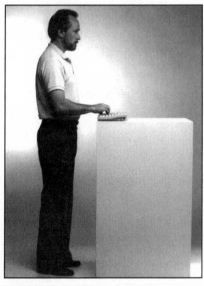

Using a keyboard with an open, erect posture.

Two simple, practical things to pay attention to are your shoes and the floor. It is especially important that your shoes fit comfortably. High heel shoes or shoes that cram your toes into a stylish point will not allow you to stand and work comfortably. Shoes should be relatively flat and should allow the bones of your feet to spread out in their natural way. It is also important that you stand on a resilient surface rather than hard concrete or tile. The floor surface should be resilient but not so soft that it interferes with good posture. (AliMed is one source for floor mats. See the Resources section at the end of Chapter 15.)

KEYBOARD PLACEMENT

Once you are standing upright, you can find your most comfortable keyboard placement. When you type, your elbows should hang naturally by your sides, with approximately a ninety degree bend, and your hands should be in the neutral semi-turned position. Wherever your hands are, there your keyboard should be.

One way of determining keyboard height is by elbow position. Stand next to the counter that will support the keyboard for standing use and turn ninety degrees, so your arm is next to the counter. Bend your elbow to ninety degrees. The home row of keys should be just slightly higher than the point of your elbow. In other words, you should be able to place your elbow on your keyboard by raising your elbow slightly. Placing the keyboard at that height will allow the easiest and most natural use of your arms.

How far from the counter should you stand? When your wrists are neutral, your fingers naturally bent, and your elbows hanging by your side, the home row of keys should fall under your fingertips. If you stand so that you don't have to reach out beyond the natural placement of your hands to get to the keyboard, you will automatically be at the right distance.

EXPERIMENT: KEYBOARD HEIGHT AND ANGLE

Try placing your keyboard on a surface four or five inches (ten or twelve centimeters) lower than the counter height just specified. Notice what your arms and hands feel like as you type on that surface. You have to bend your wrists back to adjust your hands to the keyboard, and that can cause a good deal of strain.

There is, however, a way of making a keyboard that is a few inches too low quite comfortable. If you raise the edge that is closest to you, the keyboard will angle away from you. You can adjust the angle to match the angle of your forearms as they slope downward to reach the keyboard. Since this preserves the natural line of the arms/wrists/hands, it can be quite comfortable. It is simple to put a strip of wood or a towel roll under the front edge of the keyboard.

Try putting your keyboard up too high. You will probably find that putting it too high is not as uncomfortable as putting it too low. You can put something under the rear edge of the keyboard to angle it to match the angle of your forearms. If you can maintain the semi-turned position of your hand on the keyboard, bending your elbows to an acute angle to raise your hands upward may not be too uncomfortable.

Can you vary the height of the surface on which your keyboard rests? If it is on a built-in counter, you probably cannot vary it. If the counter is low for you, then you could put a wooden board under your keyboard to raise it up. If the counter is too high for you, you could stand on one or more layers of plywood or a wooden box or something of the sort. Experiment with different keyboard heights until you find the adjustment that is most comfortable for you.

WRITING

If the work surface height is correct for your keyboard placement, you will have little difficulty with writing even though your paper documents will be lower than your keyboard. Standing balanced on your feet, you will probably position your hand on the writing surface by changing how much you bend your elbow rather than by dropping your shoulder, as you might when you sit. In addition, when you write, you turn your hand even farther into the semi-turned position than for keyboarding. In that position, moving your hand down a bit farther than the optimal writing surface height won't place any strain on your wrist.

However, your work surface height may not be correct for your keyboard placement. If it is much too high or low, you may experience difficulty with writing, and of course you will also be experiencing difficulty with keyboarding. If the surface is too low, you can write on a book or a board, and if the surface is too high, you can stand on something.

MONITOR HEIGHT

Given a good standing posture and keyboard placement, the ideal position of the monitor becomes clear. Just as in sitting, the center of the screen should be placed where your gaze happens to fall. Remember that in a normal, erect posture, your line of vision will be somewhat below the horizon, so the monitor should be lower than your eyes and tilted to meet your gaze. In addition, it should still be in front of you, about an arm's length away.

How many standing computer workstations are as adjustable as sitting workstations? You may not be able to adjust the monitor position for your needs. Also, if you are in a job where you have to deal with the public—for example, if you are a bank teller—you may not be able to position the monitor where it would be ideal. The ideal placement would put the monitor approximately in front of your face, but that would place it between you and the people you deal with. You may have to have your monitor lower than you would like or off to the side.

If your monitor is too low, you may find that you hang your head forward and down to look at it, but that movement will tend to collapse your chest. It will also tend to make you lean your shoulders back, which will arch your back. If you must live with a low monitor, rather than dropping your head, you can stand erect and rotate just your head (as was discussed in Chapter 16). If you look again at the picture of my son reading (in Chapter 4), you will see that he does just that movement to look at the book on the floor. To rotate your head, stand erect and gently raise the back of your head slightly up while moving your nose down. That movement will lengthen the back of your neck and rotate your skull down. (See the Head

Balance experiment in Chapter 9.) Remember to relax your throat and jaws.

If your monitor is too high, you may be able to stand on plywood to raise yourself up so that your monitor falls under your natural line of sight.

Try to avoid placing your monitor off to the side. That will force you to maintain a twist in your neck and torso, which could be uncomfortable and damaging over the long run. If you must work with your monitor off to one side, make sure to take frequent movement breaks. Twist to the other side and do large, whole body movements to release and relax your muscles.

REST AND MOVEMENT BREAKS

If you cannot position your monitor or keyboard to allow comfortable computer use, you must be especially careful to take rest and movement breaks. Relieving your muscles of strain and giving them a chance to rest will undo some of the effects of computer stress.

The Three-Minute Movement Breaks (Chapter 14) are appropriate for people at standing workstations. They will reduce muscle tension and improve blood flow, and since you are already standing, you could break up the movement series and do the exercises singly as five-second movement breaks. You could also adapt the Five-Second Movement Breaks (Chapter 12) to be done while standing. You can use them as brief movement breaks just to break out of a static standing posture at your computer.

However, standing workstation use often involves many elements other than just computer use, and you may already be doing so much movement that you have much less need for these movement breaks. Nonetheless, if the movements you do are not a balanced set of whole body movements, you may find these movement breaks very relaxing and energizing. In addition to doing some relaxing movements, you may also want to use some break time to get off your feet, sit down, and rest.

If you do happen to be an airline ticket agent, or you do some other job involving lots of lifting and moving, in order to avoid injuries and unnecessary fatigue, pay attention to the rules for correct lifting given in the chapter on Using Laptops (Chapter 16).

In the end, standing at a keyboard is very much like sitting at a keyboard. If you stay aware of yourself and pay attention to your workstation setup, you will be able to use your computer comfortably.

KEY POINTS

- Balance your body over its centerline, with your weight falling straight through to your feet. Don't lean your shoulders back and arch your back to counterbalance the weight of your arms when they are held out forward. Instead, move your pelvis back just a bit. Lengthen your body upward.
- Let your elbows hang comfortably by your side. Ideally you should keep your forearms horizontal and, if the counter height is correct, place the keyboard where your hands happen to be.
- Ideally, your monitor should be placed where your gaze happens to fall. If you need to place the monitor lower, don't collapse your head/neck to look down. Lengthen your body and rotate your head instead. If you must place the monitor to one side, make sure to take frequent movement breaks.

18

CHANGING THE
WORK ENVIRONMENT

There are situations in which computer users have fairly complete, direct control over their work environment. Some users are self-employed or work at home and telecommute. Other computer users are on the road a lot and can set up their workstation any way they want, within the constraints of what is available. Schools may allow teachers a lot of latitude in how they set up classroom computers. And there are companies that encourage employees to set up their workstations in whatever ways help their comfort and productivity. With the ideas and skills taught in this book, computer users can arrange their workstations to create safe and comfortable work situations.

However, there are other work situations in which people may not be given full freedom to control their work environments. Some employers might find the ideas expressed in this book new and unconvincing. It takes time for many people to adjust to the ideas that using computers can be dangerous and that employees must receive training in body awareness and workstation setup.

The key idea presented in this book is that through learning and using body awareness skills people can reduce computer stress. Rather than recommending a simple, quick equipment fix to solve the problem of Repetitive Strain Injuries (RSI), *Comfort at Your Computer* recommends encouraging employees to become self-aware and make their own decisions about what they need. This can be an especially new and strange way of thinking for many companies. It simply isn't what they are used to, and it may take time for them to come to grips with it. In every area of life, some people see and understand new ideas quickly and others take more time adjusting to change. That isn't bad. It provides a balance between conserving old ways and adopting new ways.

Many companies are still run in an older way. In one workshop I conducted, a participant told us that she worked for a company that monitored the number of keystrokes per hour. She had to type rapidly and without stopping in order to meet the company goals, and she was allowed only two brief rest breaks per day. In another workshop, a participant said that her company had strict office decor policies and was so concerned with maintaining the office aesthetics that employees were forbidden to bring in their own, more comfortable chairs. At a third workshop, I was given the name of a personnel manager at a large company and asked to phone him and talk about the work I was doing with computer users. I phoned and described it briefly, and his immediate response was, "Oh, we don't have any computer stress at our company." I suppose that's possible, but somehow I wonder whether his employees would have agreed.

Companies like these are on the edge of change. They have the scary opportunity to embrace change and become more productive. In every real business opportunity—or every real opportunity in all of life—there is risk and fear, and the idea of moving toward a very new company outlook can be very unsettling. So it may take time and thought for employers to embrace the changes.

• • • • • • •

There are two basic ideas to focus on in discussions of change. The first is that computer safety is cost effective. Greater comfort and safety will reduce fatigue, improve concentration, and improve job performance. Productivity will be increased by helping workers use computers in comfort. Not only that, but the money required for medical treatment of computer-related injuries will be reduced, and so will the money required for litigation concerning RSI and for finding and training employees to replace those who are disabled by computer work. Whatever money is spent on creating a safe workplace will be made up for in increased productivity and reduced costs.

The second idea is that it is inhumane to let people suffer and injure themselves simply because it would take some thought, effort, and money to prevent or relieve their suffering. After all, in the end, the business of business is serving *people*.

As you discuss such issues with company management, remember to use the body awareness techniques you have learned in this book to stay relaxed, caring, and strong. If you look at people as enemies, that will encourage them to feel like and act like enemies. If you remember to see them as possible allies, that will help move them toward as spirit of cooperation. Of course, there will be times when a reasonable, amicable presentation of a problem will not make a dent in closed-minded thinking. Even in those situations, you might as well stay relaxed since getting upset won't help resolve the situation and will interfere with your effective, comfortable functioning.

• • • • • • •

It is important to realize that computer users are running up against the real limits of the human body. In order to continue using computers in the workplace, the physiological limitations of the body will have to be respected. If the question is "What workstation setup will allow eight hours of uninterrupted computer work every day?" there may be no answer at all. Even correct body use and good workstation design will not prevent the effects of overuse. There really must be a balance between correct workstation setup and body use on the one hand and respect for human limits on the other. Whether employers make changes voluntarily or regulatory laws are passed, in the long run some standards covering computer and video display terminal use will undoubtedly emerge.

For the best control of RSI, there needs to be a comprehensive workplace program. The importance of RSI prevention must be stressed. If employees are simply told what to do without being convinced that it is important to do it, no great improvements will be made. There must be training programs to teach employees correct body use, correct workstation setup, and proper job design. New employees must be taught the material when they are first hired. Older employees must be taught the material as well, and periodic refresher courses are necessary to keep people focused on correct body use and job design. *Comfort at Your Computer* is designed so that computer users can master the body awareness learning they need by going through the book, and this can serve as the foundation for a workplace RSI education program.

Any RSI program must be based on the idea of giving computer users time. They must be given time to practice and learn how to use computers safely. They must also be encouraged to work at a pace that is safe and to take rest and movement breaks, even if that means that they actually do produce less in the short run. Of course, in the long run, computer users will be more productive if they can avoid RSI difficulties.

In order to make sure that body awareness and workstation setup information is actually utilized by employees, there must be ways of monitoring employee work patterns. Needless to say, to gain employee acceptance and participation, such training and monitoring programs should be set up as cooperative, rather than coercive, measures.

The most important element in dealing with RSI is prevention, but monitoring RSI incidences and providing proper medical treatment and follow-up body and movement awareness education will also be important. Once RSI has been identified and treated, changes will have to be made in the workplace to prevent re-injuries. Doing the same thing the same way will lead to re-occurrence of the same injuries.

An overall survey of the work done in the company and the incidence of RSI associated with various tasks and workstations will offer a good starting place in reducing RSI risks. Significant employee absences or productivity decreases may point to workstation discomfort and developing RSI's. It will be important to get subjective information from the employees about elements of stress and discomfort.

It will be important to have systematic procedures for early identification of developing RSI problems in employees. The earlier that problems are identified and interventions instituted, the less costly and injurious the problems will be. Employees and supervisors should be educated about early signs of discomfort and developing RSI's, and there should be a systematic way for employees to get help to prevent problems from worsening. If employees do develop discomfort or actual RSI, their needs must be met sympathetically and supportively. If that does not happen, employees will feel increased stress, which will in turn worsen the RSI problem.

If time and money are not invested in preventing RSI's, then even more time and money will be invested in treating the problems. Structuring the company so that people pay attention to proper job design, proper workstation set up, good interpersonal atmosphere, proper body use, and proper movement breaks will be the best long term solution to the problem of how to use computers safely and comfortably.

KEY POINTS

- Computer users are running up against the real limits of the human body. In order to continue using computers in the workplace, the physiological limitations of the body will have to be respected.
- For the best control of RSI, there needs to be a comprehensive RSI training program that will emphasize correct body use, proper equipment choices, correct workstation setup, proper job design, and RSI monitoring.

19

THE BEGINNING

This is not the end. It is the beginning. Now that you have thought through and tried out new ways of moving and working, you have the opportunity to keep on experimenting, learning, and improving. Computers will be with us for a long time. Whatever changes they may undergo, and whatever changes your work may undergo, you can be sure that the basic nature of human movement and awareness will stay the same. You will be able to apply the basic principles of body and movement awareness and keep getting more and more comfortable as you work.

KEY CONCEPTS FOR COMFORT AT YOUR COMPUTER

The concepts and exercises covered in *Comfort at Your Computer* can be summarized briefly. As you read through the following list, can you recall the full body of information hinted at by the summary points?

1—Working at a computer for long hours is an intense and strenuous athletic event. You need both *proper equipment and proper body use*. Knowing your body is the key to effective movement technique, proper equipment selection, and correct workstation setup.

2—Every element of your mind/body is connected to every other element of your mind/body. What you do in one part of your self influences what you do in your whole self. Mind, body, movement, computer, physical work environment, and interpersonal work environment all form an *interlocking, interconnected, interdependent system*.

3—Noticing *what you feel in your body* as you work at the computer is the key to detecting problems, reducing discomfort, and preventing injuries. Paying attention to sensations of strain, compression, tension, constriction, and fatigue will allow you to make changes. Noticing the sensations of dynamic and static action will help you understand your movements.

4—You can learn to *use your body well*:

- Relax and open your pelvis, belly, chest, and throat.
- Align your pelvis, spinal column, and head for balanced, relaxed stability.
- Breathe softly and fully, letting your belly and chest expand gently as you inhale.
- Use your shoulders, arms, and hands in a neutral, relaxed, well-supported fashion.
- Position your legs in a free, supportive manner to achieve a good foundation for your whole body.
- Use your eyes in a relaxed, soft way.
- Maintain your body in a lengthened alignment. Balance your body along its center line, and use your pelvis as the core of your body and movement.

5—*Keep moving!* Take rest breaks, and take movement breaks. Vary the tasks you work at.

6—*Arrange your workstation* to support your body in your position of comfort and efficiency. Make sure your chair, desk, input devices, and monitor are all adjusted and positioned to conform to your body dimensions.

7—Discovering how to use computers in comfort is an ongoing *process of learning*. Getting compulsive about perfection will itself be stressful and will undermine your learning and change. It is important to give yourself the gift of patience and continuing curiosity. Enjoying the process of investigation will make it easier to continue learning.

8—Opening this book once in a while and *going through the exercises again* will help you refresh your memory of them and make sure you are still using them in your everyday work.

Once you have experienced and understood what these concepts refer to, they can seem pretty simple. But they are very important and very far reaching. Paying attention to yourself as you use your computer will completely change how you work.

From the exercises in this book, you have learned how to work in comfort. Much of the material in this book can be absorbed by many people very quickly. One of the people who read an early draft of this book is a writer and had had a lot of back pain as she worked at her computer. She told me that after reading the book, she no longer hurt when she worked. I've had people tell me that after learning this material, they reorganized their whole work environment and achieved amazing comfort.

I've also had people tell me that understanding and learning body material that was new for them was difficult. If you do run into difficulties, try to keep a positive outlook. What we are talking about in this book is at once simple and complex. Your body and movement patterns are part of your fundamental identity, and changing yourself on such a fundamental level may take some time. Beyond that, some of what you have experienced in this book is contrary to our culture's norms for correct body use, and swimming against the tide can take some effort.

You will find that continuing to work on self-awareness will be worth the effort. Attaining comfort will be worth some effort and some patience.

You can do it. In all of human history, this is the first time millions of people have spent millions of hours working on computers. It's not surprising that we all make some mistakes. But with what you have learned, you will be able to spot your mistakes and use them as springboards to solutions. You will be able to achieve *Comfort at Your Computer.*

WORKSHOPS AND CONSULTATIONS

I offer workshops and private lessons in body awareness and computer use and also serve as a consultant for workstation design and setup. Many people find live teaching very helpful as an addition to printed material. Some people find it quicker and easier to absorb body learning when it is provided live, since they don't have to bridge from the intellectual process of reading to the kinesthetic process of body feeling. Having a teacher present allows people to ask about the unique aspects of their body use and movement and unique aspects of their jobs and workstation setups. In addition, learning the material in a group setting with a teacher present can be more enjoyable and more motivating.

A very different reason for attending a workshop is to learn how to help employees use this book and learn how to work comfortably and safely at their computers. People who are setting up a program in safe computer use at their company, school, or other organization would find it helpful to experience the workshop and observe how the material is taught and how people respond to it.

For Information about *Comfort at Your Computer* seminars, contact:
Paul Linden, Ph.D.
Columbus Center for Movement Studies
221 Piedmont Road
Columbus, OH 43214 USA

Voice & Fax: (614) 262-3355
E-mail: paullinden@aol.com
Website: http://www.being-in-movement.com

QUESTIONS AND COMMENTS

I am constantly working to improve both the content and presentation of the *Comfort at Your Computer* training, and if you would like to contact me with ideas about the book, I would appreciate hearing from you. If you have any questions about, or difficulties with, the book, any problems or equipment that should be covered but weren't, or any suggestions or success stories, I would be very interested in hearing about them. (However, I may not be able to offer advice about individual problems.)

I will try to respond to letters. But if I get swamped with mail, I might not be able to. If I don't respond to *your* note, please don't take it personally. I may have reached the physiological limit for human computer use and be out in the sun, taking my own advice about not overworking.

Whether I respond or not, thank you for your interest and effort in dropping me a note.

You can reach me at:

Paul Linden, Ph.D.

Columbus Center for Movement Studies

221 Piedmont Road

Columbus, OH 43214 USA

Voice & Fax: (614) 262-3355

E-Mail: paullinden@aol.com

Website: http://www.being-in-movement.com

Appendix ⟮C⟯

BIOGRAPHY

As a body awareness educator, I am interested in the human dimension of information. When I read books, I always want to know a little something about the *person* behind the information and how they learned what they are writing about. So here is a brief statement of who I am and how I came to learn the material I teach.

The material in *Comfort at Your Computer* comes from thirty years of body and movement awareness practice. It wasn't until after college that I began my life as a mover. Before that I was a philosophy major (which you could probably tell). What I was most interested in was figuring out how people develop their philosophies of life. Even in high school, I had the feeling that our philosophies come from something about the way we are *built*, though I didn't know then how true it is that physical structure is the foundation for mental functioning.

Shortly after college, I happened to see a film of Morihei Ueshiba, the founder of Aikido, demonstrating the art. Something in me knew that Aikido was a practical way of doing in my body things that up until then I had only thought about. I started Aikido and have been practicing it ever since. My emphasis on relaxation, power, and balance stems primarily from my practice of Aikido.

Aikido is intensely physical and demands being fully present in your experience of the movements. As I practiced Aikido, I began to get in

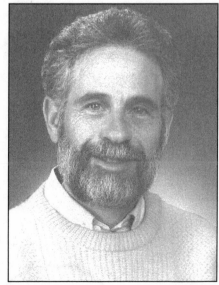

touch with how intellectual I was and how little I was aware of my body. However, Aikido is very non-intellectual, and it didn't offer me any bridge for moving from my intellect to my body and actually mastering the kinds of movement Aikido requires.

I found that the only way I could become aware of my body and improve my movement was to create, on my own, detailed experiments to focus on my breathing, muscle use, posture, balance, and so on. I found a way to use the intellect in the service of body awareness. That was the beginning of the kind of teaching contained in this book. I continued practicing Aikido and achieved a black belt in that. I practiced yoga, took lessons in Alexander work, became a Feldenkrais® instructor, and earned a black belt in Karate. Along the way, I earned my M.A. and Ph.D. in Physical Education. All the while, I was concentrating on developing a mind/body teaching approach that fused an intellectual and experimental process with body and movement awareness experience.

Over the years of studying my own body and movement, I developed many movement awareness experiments and a set of fundamental movement principles. When I began teaching Aikido, I used that material to supplement the Aikido and help my students gain the body awareness necessary for learning the art. It happened that people who were not Aikidoists began showing up at my door inquiring about body awareness training as it applied to their areas of concern. More and more of my teaching was outside Aikido, and I became a somatic educator without ever meaning to. I've worked with people on topics ranging from stress management and conflict resolution, to athletic or musical performance, to recovery from child abuse. I've helped people redesign workstations, and I patented a new form of bicycle handlebars designed to provide greater structural ease and power. Underneath all the diversity is a unity. It's all about balance and wholeness—the development of awareness, power, and compassion.

I call the teaching process I have developed *Being In Movement*® mindbody training. If you would like a broader description of it than this book includes, you might be interested in the following papers (most of which are downloadable from my website, http://www.being-in-movement.com):

"Being In Movement: Intention as a Somatic Meditation," *Somatics*, Autumn, 1988.

"Applications of Being In Movement in Working with Incest Survivors," *Somatics*, Autumn, 1990.

"Developing Power and Sensitivity through Movement Awareness Training," *American Music Teacher*, October, 1992.

"Body Awareness, Critical Thinking and Self-Scrutiny," *Inquiry*, Parts I and II, November, 1993 and February, 1994.

"Somatic Literacy: Bringing Somatic Education Into Physical Education," *Journal of Physical Education, Recreation and Dance*, September, 1994.

"Too Much of a Good Thing: Prevention of Computer-Related Repetitive Strain Injuries Among Children," *Technological Horizons in Education Journal*, August, 1998.

"Embodying Power and Love: A Somatic Approach to Understanding Violence and Teaching Peace," *Perspective (Association of Humanistic Psychology)*, December, 1999.

INDEX

Aikido, 161, 295
AliMed catalog, 253
Anger, 89, 91, 211
Armrests See Chair: armrests
Arms,
  positioning, 99-101, 104-106
  standing balance, 282
  support by body, 93-96, 98
Attention See also Intention
Attention, 20, 31

Back, 87, 282
Balance, 52, 58
Being In Movement training, 22,
  296
Belly, 51-53, 59, 62, 64, 87
Bifocals, 147
Blood pump See Muscle: as blood
  pump
Blood pump, 33, 118, 158
Blood vessels, entrapment, 35
Body awareness, 5-6, 13-23, 30, 33,
  67, 118, 161
Body core, 51
Body image See also Culture
Body image, 52, 53-59, 80, 90
Body use See Posture
Books 13, 23, 159, 228, 247, 252
Breathing, 16, 30, 51, 61-66, 69, 87
  exercise, 61, 64, 68, 110, 194, 196
Carpal tunnel syndrome, 36
Catalogs, 252
Centered sitting See also Posture:
  optimal, See also Sitting: cen-
  tered style

Centered sitting, 80, 82, 157
Centering, 66, 84, 89, 125
Chair, 213-221
  armrests, 158, 220
  backrest, 157, 218
  height, 214
  kneeling, 159, 217
  padding, 217
  seat pan, 216, 218
  secretary's chair, 219
  stool, 220
  wheels, 219
Chest, 87, 90-91, 98
  elevation, 87, 131, 155
Children 3, 45, 223, 245, 297
Children, 58, 62
Clothes, 52, 111
Company See Work environment:
  corporate
Compassion See also Heart
Compassion, 88, 91
Compression, 32, 51, 59, 60
Computer stress See also Stress
Computer stress, 3, 25, 28-48, 91
  causes, 38-47
  costs, 29
  effects, 28-29, 34-36, 137
  prevention, 4, 48
  social effects, 29
  treatment, 4
Connection See also Holism,
  Mind/body
Connection, 16, 20, 28, 52, 89, 160
Cranz, Galen 159
Culture See also Body image

Culture, 51, 53-59, 80, 90, 117, 131, 155, 160-161
Desk, 221-225, 247
 floor, 225
 for writing, 223-224
 height, 221-223, 236
Desktop workstation, 209-252
 resources, 252
Diaphragm, 62
Dictation (See Voice)
Digitizing (see Graphics tablet)
Disks, intervertebral, 34, 123, 154
Drawing, 234, 238
Dynamic action, 33
Elbows, 100, 105
Electromyography, 20
Emotional strain, 27
Emotions See also Feelings
Emotions, 67
Entrapment, 35
Environment See Work environ-
 ment
Equipment, 10, 212
Exercise See also Experiment,
 Practice
 proper attitude, 8-9
Exercise,
 pacing, 7
 proper attitude, 14, 15, 88, 289
Experiment See also Exercise
Experiment, 6, 13
Experimental attitude, 9
Eyes See also Monitor: technical
 characteristics
Eyes,
 aiming, 141
 focusing, 139-140
 glasses, 147
 lighting, 144-146
 lubrication, 138
 position, 131, 133, 151
 relaxation, 146, 148-151, 177, 247
 strain, 137, 142, 146
 structure & function, 138-147
Face, 134
Fatigue, 34, 35, 95, 146

Fear, 91
Fear/startle response See also
 Fight-or-flight
Fear/startle response, 63
Feeling the body See Body
 awareness
Feelings See also Emotions,
 Centering
Feelings, 21, 67, 88, 89, 146
 negative, 66, 89, 90-91
Feet, 109
Feldenkrais Method 23, 168
Feldenkrais Method, 176
Fight-or-flight
 See also Fear/startle response 63
Fight-or-flight, 61
Flexibility See Stretching
Floor, 225, 286
Furniture selection, 5
Gallwey, Timothy 13
Glare, 145
Glasses, 147
Global Computer Supplies catalog,
 253
Grandjean, Etienne, 252
Graphics tablet 234
Graphics tablet, 239
 body use, 238
 desk height, 236
 hand use, 237
 position, 235-236
Graphics, 42
Hand position, half-turned See
 Hands:neutral
Hands, 96-101, 236, 237
 neutral position, 98, 104
 on mouse, 232
 orientation, 98-101
Handwriting recognition, 234
Hardware, 10
Head, 129
 balance, 129-133
 position, 151
 reading movements, 248-249
 relaxation, 134
 rotation, 132, 288

Health, 9
Heart, 88, See also Compassion
High heels, 117, 215
Hips, 78, 112, 122
Holism, 7, See also Connection, 16, 22
Iliac crest, 112, 173
Iliacus muscle, 78, 81, 157
Imbalance See also Balance
Imbalance, 32, 90
Injury, 17, 21
Input devices, 225-239
  keyboard, 225
  mouse, 231-232
  trackball, 233
Intention, 18, 20
Interpersonal relations, 91
Ischial tuberosities See Sitbones
Jacobson, Edmund, 20
Job demands, 43
Job design, 41
Keyboard position, 100, 225
  distance, 104
  height, 287
  orientation, 226
  slant, 105, 227-228, 287
  with laptop, 255
  with standing workstation, 286-287
Keyboard, 101, 225-230, 266
  feel, 228
  V-shaped, 229
Keyboarding See Typing
Knaster, Mirka 23
Knees, 113
Laptop,
  built-in trackball, 266-267
  carrying cases, 268-271
  carrying, 277-278
  lifting briefcase, 273
  lifting shoulder bag or knapsack, 274
  lifting, 123, 267-268, 272
  on an airplane, 265-266
  problems, 255-257
  with a chair, 258, 261
  without a chair, 261-264

Learning See Exercise: proper attitude
Legs
  relaxation, 111
Legs, 109, 224
  movements, 176
  position, 115, 116
  relaxation, 109
  standing, 282
  support, 112-124
  use in lifting, 272, 273
Lengthening 66, 69
Lengthening, 103, 133, 172, 185, 200, 277
Lifestyle, 9, 40, 257
Lifting See Laptop: lifting
Lighting, 144-146, 250
Limpness, 32, 51, 56, 59-61
Lumbar support, 157, 216, 219
Macros, 239
Micromovement, 20
Mind/body See also Connection, Holism
Mind/body, 16, 20, 32, 89
Mirror, 247
Monitor See also Laptop, screen
Monitor, 240-247
  position, 131, 243-245, 247, 288
  radiation, 242-243
  stand, 245, 247
  technical characteristics, 240-241
  text characteristics, 241-242
Mouse, 231-232
  for drawing, 238
Movement breaks,
  at the computer, 165
  for home, 181-196
  for the office, 200-206
Movement,
  effective, 4, 5
  job requirements, 42
  process, 14, 15, 31, 33
Muscle, 30, 32
  as blood pump, 33, 118
  fatigue, 34, 213
  tension, 16
  work, 153, 213

Neck, 129
Nerves, 20
Nerves, entrapment 35
Opening See Lengthening
Palms See Hands
Paper documents, 248-252
  head movements, 248-249
  lighting, 250
  read-only documents, 248
  stand, 250
  write-on documents, 223, 236,
    251
Paper,
  read-only documents,
Pascarelli, Emil, 228
Pelvic floor muscles, 62, 80
Pelvis, 73, 83, 94, 112, 216, 283
  forward/backward, 76
  rotation, 76-77, 78, 79, 94, 116,
    119, 272
Pheasant, Stephen, 252
Postural strain, 27, 95
Posture, 16, 35, 39, 73, 130
  optimal, 58, 62, 71-72, 80, 95,
    105, 112, 114, 115, 122, 124,
    151, 153-154
Posture, optimal See also
  Sitting:centered style
Practice, 6
Pressure & irritation, 106
Pressure, on body parts, 35, 213,
    214
Psoas muscle, 78, 157
Quilter, Deborah, 228
QWERTY keyboard, 226
Ramazzini, Bernardino, 252
Relaxation, 33, 59-60, 183
  belly, 51, 52, 64
  eyes, 146, 148-151
  hands, 96
  head, 134
  legs, 109-110
  pelvic musculature, 51

Repetitive Strain Injury, 28, 293
  medical treatment, 10, 228
  workplace program, 293-294
Resources, 22, 228, 252
Rest breaks See also Movement
  breaks
Rest breaks, 43, 166, 199-200
Schools (see Children)
Scope, 9-11
Seat pan, 76, 159, 216-217, 218
Shoes, 111, 117, 215, 225, 286
Shoulder girdle, 94, 236
Sitbones, 80
Sitting "straight", 78, 80, 88, 131
Sitting,
  centered style, 80, 155
  half-standing style, 159, 217
  reclining style, 157, 158, 216
  slumping, 76, 114
  straight up style, 155-157
  straightening up, 76
  with towel support, 82, 218
Somatic education, 22
SOREHAND, 253
Speaking (See Voice)
Spinal Column, 34, 73, 87, 94, 119,
    133, 153
Standing posture, 284
Standing workstation, 281
  keyboard position, 286-287
  monitor position, 288
  posture, 281-285
Static action, 33-35, 141
Strain, 95, 142
Stress, 22, See also Computer
  stress, 25-28, 38, 48
  emotional, 40
  identifying, 30, 32
  postural, 39
Stress-related illness, 26, 28
Stressor, 25
  physical, 27
  psychological, 27

Stretching, 167, 182-184
  exercises 177, 181-193
Students (see Children)
Talking (See Voice)
Telephone, 42, 239
Tension, 16, 21, 32, 51, 55, 59
TIFAQ, 253
Towel support, 82, 218
Trackball, 233
Typing, 100
Ulnar flexion, 100, 103
Verticality, 71, 80
Voice 68-69, 239
Voice Recognition 68, 239

Walking, 52, 110, 120
Wanting See also Intention
Wanting, 18
Website, 253, 296
Work environment,
  corporate, 46-47, 291
  interpersonal, 44
  physical 10
  physical, 44
Wrist supports, 158, 230
Wrists, 36, 101, 102-103
  stretches, 177
  ulnar flexion, 100
Writing, 223, 236, 287